The American Diet:
A Recipe for Disaster

We Are What We Eat, Drink and Breathe

Edmund Devroey, M.D.

Foreword by
Professor G.N. Schrauzer, Ph.D., F.A.C.N., C.N.S.

Health Balance, LLC
San Diego, California

Cover design by Catherine Devriese and Helen Bertels
Book design by Joyce L'Heureux and Debra Spann
Edited by Mo Rafael

This book is not intended as a substitute for the recommendations of physicians or other health-care providers. Rather, it is intended to offer information to help the reader, in cooperation with physicians and health professionals, in a joint quest for optimum health.

Edmund Devroey, MD
The American Diet: A Recipe for Disaster
Includes bibliographical references
ISBN 0-9765613-0-1

Printed in the United States of America
By Delta Printing Solutions
First edition, April 2005
Library of Congress Control Number: 2005921484
Publisher: Health Balance, LLC
e-mail: sec@healthbalance.net

To Mieke

Foreword

While great progress was achieved in the U.S. during the past half century in nearly every branch of science and technology, in the field of nutrition we Americans did not do so well. Obesity has risen to epidemic proportions along with alarming increases in the incidence of diabetes and steadily climbing death rates from heart disease. What can be done to halt and reverse these trends? We must change the way we eat. This well-researched book spells out for a broad readership what is wrong with the average American diet and how it must be changed to improve our health and productivity. Its author is a Belgian-born physician who realized that he could achieve superior therapeutic results by correcting the poor eating habits of his patients. After he arrived in the United States he joined my research group at the University of California, San Diego, where he participated in groundbreaking studies of essential trace elements. This experience furthered his interest in the role of nutrition in health and disease and prompted him to write this book. I recommend this book to all who are seeking concise, up-to-date information on diet and health fundamentals as well as some of the most recent advances in the field of nutrition.

Gerhard Norbert Schrauzer, Ph.D., F.A.C.N., C.N.S.

Acknowledgments

I thank the associates of the company American Longevity for the thousands of e-mails they sent requesting nutritional guidelines for themselves and their customers. The questions and concerns expressed in their messages have had a great influence in determining the thrust of this book and the content of each chapter. Marianne Gordon was the meticulous proofreader of the original manuscript. Mo Rafael was the diligent and skillful editor of the current book. She trimmed down my overly detailed descriptions and translated my "French-speak" into conventional English. Joyce L'Heureux and Debra Spann shaped the interior design. My wife Mieke was my ever-dependable final proofreader. The cover design and the CD label is by Catherine Devriese and her friend Helen Bertels. The picture on the cover is by Paul Bowers. My thanks also to Steve Haskins, Ned Ardagna and Sidney Goldman for their advice, legal and otherwise.

Contents

Introduction

The American Diet: A Recipe for Disaster is a provocative title, is it not? Intentionally so. This book is a wake-up call to Americans, and I make no apologies for what may feel like a brusque awakening. I believe that we must become aware of the errors in our way of eating and in the way we think about—or do not think about—our diet. Our health as individuals and as a nation depends upon it.

Attention Americans!

How can something "American" be a "disaster"? The term *American* elicits strong positive beliefs. What is American is considered to be inherently good, even the best in the world. Americans swear by all things American. By contrast, the term *disaster* has a truly un-American ring to it. It defines a happening that causes great harm and damage. A disaster is a serious misfortune, a calamity.

I have purposely juxtaposed these terms for two reasons: to grab your attention and to throw down the gauntlet. In this book I challenge the average American diet because of its direct connection with poor health. The purpose of this book is to help you understand why it deserves to be questioned and how you can make vital changes in your own diet. Please take note of the following clarification. By "the American diet" I mean all that we Americans eat and drink on an everyday basis. I am not referring to special diets created for a specific purpose.

This book lays out the imbalances in our American diet.

It analyzes and discusses their impact on our health. It also promotes the understanding of how we can change unhealthy eating habits to healthy ones.

Hard Scientific Evidence

The American Diet: A Recipe for Disaster contains hard scientific evidence. This scientific evidence comes from the growing number of publications describing the links between diet excesses and deficiencies and human health. Over the last 5 years the number of these publications has been increasing at an accelerated rate. The Scirus search engine[1] yields 8,568 such documents issued in the four year period from 1991 through 1994 and 435,897—fifty times more—over a similar period of time from 2001 through 2004.

The errors that have shaped the American diet and their impact on the health of the Americans will be brought to light only when this scientific research becomes public knowledge. May this book be an instrument of it.

About the Author

First Practice in Africa

After graduating from the University of Louvain Medical School in Belgium in 1952, I had the opportunity to serve as a volunteer in the Belgian Congo (now Zaire). As a young medical doctor I welcomed the challenges of such an experience. I went to Congo and was assigned to a rural hospital in the middle of nowhere.

My patients were exclusively natives from villages in the surrounding area who presented with various ailments.

Some of them, mostly young children, were so thin they looked as if they were severely undernourished. Yet food was plentiful and they were eating well. Their bodies were thin everywhere except for swollen bellies and edema of the lower extremities. The cause of their condition was intestines full of worms and parasites that deprived them of the nourishment from most of the food they ingested. These individuals were so debilitated that even a minimal health challenge was for them a life-threatening condition.

Although witnessing people dying from the sheer exhaustion of debilitation was a sight that I would not forget, little did I realize at the time how this experience in Africa would come to completely and forever influence my view of medicine. **The limitations of the medical model in treating diseases (in this case, the intestinal worms and parasites) had been exposed. The primary importance of nutrition and intestinal absorption for health were made crystal clear to me.**

Fellowship in Ob-Gyn and Private Practice

After my stay in Africa, I started a fellowship in Gynecology and Obstetrics at the University of Brussels Medical School. I then maintained a successful private practice in Belgium for more than 30 years. While monitoring pregnancies and delivering babies, I could not forget the children I had seen suffering and sometimes dying from malnutrition in Africa.

I started inquiring about the diet of my patients, making comments and giving them nutritional advice. Most pregnant women in my practice had started taking vitamin and mineral supplements as soon as they noticed they were pregnant.

Some of them, notwithstanding their supplementation, had premature babies and babies with intrauterine growth retardation. This was in contradiction to the accepted idea that supplementing the pregnant woman's diet with vitamins and minerals was the best guaranty for a successful outcome. I became interested in finding out if starting the supplementation with minerals and vitamins before pregnancy would provide even greater benefits. It did, and I published the results of my observations at the 8th Congress of Perinatalogy in 1982.[2] Now it appeared I had some further work cut out for me, and it clearly revolved around nutrition.

Continuing My Education

To compensate for the lack of nutrition education in my medical school curriculum I had to educate myself. I collected all the books I could find on the subject and subscribed to several journals. The more I learned the more apparent it became that what we eat, drink and breathe has a determining impact on our health. *We Are What We Eat, Drink and Breathe* eventually became my slogan.

A Research Group on Hormones

Meanwhile, Dr. Jacques Hertoghe, other colleagues and I had created a physician research group to investigate the clinical signs of hormone deficiency. Our group was particularly interested in trying to solve the quandary surrounding thyroid hormone investigation as seen in the discrepancy between the results of lab tests and the results of physical examination. Indeed, it was the clinical experience of the members of our group that many of the patients presenting symptoms of and having complaints compatible with thyroid hormone deficiency had received conflicting lab results that showed their thyroid hormones to be within normal range.

To help solve the problem, the physicians of the group were advocating the basal temperature test promoted by Dr. Broda Barnes, and my good friend Jacques Hertoghe came up with and fine tuned a 24-hour urine thyroid hormone test. This hormone utilization test did correlate better with the clinical signs of thyroid hormone deficiency. Jacques and I were invited to lecture about our findings in Belgium, France, the Netherlands and the U.S.

Back to Nutrition

In the late 1970s our research on thyroid hormone acquired a sudden and unexpected nutritional twist. It was discovered that the trace element selenium is essential for thyroid hormone utilization. Without sufficient selenium in the diet people cannot utilize the thyroid hormone they produce. They present signs of thyroid hormone deficiency. They are functionally hypothyroid and the thyroid hormone their bodies produce but cannot use remains in their blood circulation, yielding normal results on their lab tests.[3]

An Academic Boost

The nutritional aspects of our research on hormones put me in touch with the renowned researcher Professor Gerhard N. Schrauzer who is considered to be the world expert on selenium. He offered me a postdoctoral fellowship that allowed me to join his research group at the University of California, San Diego. The research I was able to do under his direction contributed enormously to my understanding of the role of nutrition in human health and remains a highlight of my life. His encouragement greatly helped me to take my studies to the next level and to complete this book.

Full Time Research and Nutritional Advice

Research on nutrition and health is now my full-time business. I became a member of the scientific advisory board of several food supplement companies in the U.S. and abroad.

One of my actual tasks for these companies is to answer the questions concerning health and food supplements from their associates and from their consumers. A constant flow of e-mail comes from the U.S., from Australia, Canada, New Zealand, United Kingdom, Denmark and other countries. I have been answering these questions for more than six years now.

Helping People Educate Themselves

It is my experience that, because of the growing public interest in maintaining good health by supplementing the diet, many people are trying to educate themselves about nutrition and health. They do it out of necessity as they are met with indifference and ignorance and denial on the part of the medical world. (Do you know of any medical clinic where in-patients routinely receive food supplements?)

To provide my correspondents with the knowledge that they are looking for I have gradually expanded my answers to include the medical and biochemical data relevant to each topic in question. I have prepared answers to frequently asked questions and to these I have added lists of references, mostly URLs of web sites of interest. This book is a compendium of all these explanations, answers, data, references and recommendations provided as a single resource.

About this Book

The American Diet: A Recipe for Disaster is intended as a template for people willing to educate themselves about nutrition and health. It is intended to be a thorough primer, establishing the all-important links between diet and health. Although this book covers a wide variety of the kinds of health conditions that my correspondents inquire about, it intentionally differs greatly from other books that address various aspects of health and disease. Rather than advising people to blindly follow directions, *The American Diet* contains an abundance of facts, presents the conclusions at which I have arrived, and invites the reader to draw upon these facts to form new understandings for their own benefit.

Three Objectives

My objectives in writing the book are to create awareness of the connection between diet and health, to furnish arguments for the legitimacy of that connection and to provide an easy access to the scientific data supporting that connection.

1. Awareness of the Diet/Health Connection

My first objective is to raise awareness about the vital connection between diet and health. I have found that many people still daily underestimate or disregard the importance of this connection. Even those who are adept at managing their diet do not always realize the depth and the variety of the connections between diet and health. And this says nothing of the people who simply are not conscious of the connection. I want to make it clear that even a modest awareness will create big health payoffs.

2. Acceptance of the Legitimacy of Diet Correction

The second objective of this book is to convince the reader that a correct diet is one of the primary and major factors in improving and promoting health. This idea is still foreign to the medical establishment. Health practitioners are educated to use pharmaceuticals to treat the symptoms of conditions, even if these conditions result primarily, if not exclusively, from errors in the diet of their patients.

3. Accessibility of Scientific Data

The third objective is to make scientific data concerning diet and health accessible to everyone. Until about ten years ago scientific information about nutrition, like most scientific information, remained sequestered in specialized journals. The general public had little or no access to it. Over the last several years that situation has changed dramatically. While scientists still publish their articles in specialized journals, their knowledge, opinions and discoveries now also appear on web pages that are available to everyone with a World Wide Web (WWW) connection.

Nowadays the problem is no longer the availability of data but the overwhelming abundance of it. This problem is exacerbated by the fact that scientific journals and scientists are not the only ones who create web pages that address medical, scientific and health implication issues. People with limited and/or inaccurate understanding of diet can and do create web sites with a scientific guise in order to sell their products and remedies, give advice or promulgate their opinions. It is becoming increasingly difficult to know what information is accurate and to differentiate between valid and scientifically bogus web sites. Beyond that there looms the question of how best to apply the information to oneself. **Given the magnitude of these challenges it is clear that anyone in search of the most accurate nutrition information requires either a solid scientific background or a trustworthy guide.**

I offer this book to you as a trustworthy guide. It is my sincere desire that it significantly contribute to your understanding of the many connections between your diet and your health. May you learn that the essential key to improving your health is as near at hand as your willingness to learn why and how to make corrections in your daily diet.

The CD

This book comes with a CD. The CD lists the references cited in the book. But it does much more than that for the reader who has a World Wide Web connection. By clicking on the URLs in the reference list from the CD you have access to the text of the abstracts cited and for several of the references you will also have access to the full text of the publication as well as access to illustrations.

Furthermore, the CD also contains a list of more than 1,250 addresses of web sites of interest. This list is alphabetic by topic. It greatly expands the scope of information available to you and all of it is only a few clicks away.

To open some of the web pages listed in the CD you need the Adobe Reader software. If you do not already have it, Adobe Acrobat Reader is available for download free of charge at *http://www.adobe.com/products/acrobat/readstep.htm*.

Chapter 1

Life is Adaptation to Change

What is constant in life is change. For any living organism, the ability to adapt to alterations in its environment is essential in order for it to stay alive and to prosper. It is true for all organisms that only when they are in balance with their environment can they maintain life and prosper. Should the environment change or should there be an alteration in their living conditions, organisms have no other option than to adapt to the change, suffer from it or disappear.

This book has been introduced to the reader as an investigation of the connection between diet and health. So why on earth does it open with a chapter entitled "Life is Adaptation to Change"? For a very important reason—and one that we "conveniently" overlook: diet itself is a critical part of the environment of any group of organisms. A change in the fundamental composition of the organisms' diet **is** an alteration in the environment in which those organisms live. They have no choice other than to adapt to or suffer from those changes in their living conditions. But what is required to make the necessary adaptation? This, indeed, the question.

Successful Adaptation

An example of successful adaptation to an environmental change is the adaptation of bacteria to antibiotics. To us, the success of bacteria in developing a resistance to our antibiotics has been surprising. Indeed, it has become a matter of real chagrin and consternation to us as well. But it should not be a surprise because their success is nothing more than a classic example of life evolution, the consequence of successful adaptation.

Antibiotics alter the environment in which bacteria live. Bacteria adapt to antibiotics as they have adapted to other environmental changes over millions of years. Without successful adaptation to changes in their environment bacteria would have disappeared long ago.

More than 150 antibiotics have been used to attack bacteria. Each antibiotic has, over time, been rendered useless. Using successful survival strategies honed over countless generations, bacteria have learned to adapt to the introduction of one antibiotic after another into their environment. The result is the proliferation of antibiotic-resistant strains of bacteria.

How Do Bacteria Adapt to Antibiotics?

A recent and dramatic example of bacterial adaptation to environmental changes is the resistance that the bacterium *Staphylococcus aureus* has developed against the antibiotic Vancomycine. Various strains of this bacterium had developed resistance to other antibiotics, and until recently Vancomycine was the antibiotic to which no strains were resistant. Hence, it was the antibiotic of last resort used against the deadly hospital-acquired infection by the antibiotic-resistant strains of *Staphylococcus aureus*.[4]

Vancomycine kills *Staphylococcus aureus* by punching holes in the outermost layer that protects the bacteria. This layer is even exterior to the cell membrane and is referred to as "the wall." In the maintenance and repair process that *S. aureus* normally undergoes, parts of this wall of *S. aureus* are continually removed and replaced. Vancomycine can attach to the wall during the repair process and block it. A hole in the wall is lethal for the bacteria. The attachment of Vancomycine occurs only to a very specific constituent (one particular amino acid) of the wall. The bacteria that resist Vancomycine have learned to make their wall without that specific amino acid. Without that attachment site the Vancomycine can no longer launch its attack on the bacteria.

The adaptation of bacteria to environmental changes— such as the appearance of an antibiotic in their environment—is achieved via a few simple yet elegant processes: mutation, fusion/ recombination, and selection of the genes. In bacteria, as in all living organisms, changes in the genes occur during the reproduction process only.

Repetition is the Essence of the Process

Adaptation is a very incremental process. It occurs bit by bit. One thousand successive little bits may yield a useful change in the genes. This is why it takes about one thousand generations for bacteria to develop resistance to an antibiotic. Incremental repetition is the essence of the process.

Bacteria divide rapidly. In optimal conditions they may grow almost three generations in one hour. (See Table 1.) With only three generations in one day, a one-year exposure to an antibiotic may be a sufficient period of time for the bacteria to develop resistance to it.

Temp. In °F	Replication time in min.	Temp. In °F	Replication time in min.
114	32	86	33
111	22	79	56
104	21	72	96
100	22	64	260
93	28	57	400

Table 1. Replication time of *E. coli* at various temperatures. Adapted from Ingraham (1958)

Human Adaptation

An example of human adaptation to the environment is the darkening in human skin color from northern Europe to southern Africa. It is an adaptation of the skin to the sun's ultraviolet radiation that is much stronger in the tropics.

Ultraviolet (UV) rays penetrating human skin help make vitamin D, but UV rays also destroy the vitamin folic acid that is essential for reproduction. In the tropics the human skin adaptation of taking on more pigmentation protects against folic acid destruction while still allowing a sufficient penetration of UV rays to make vitamin D. In higher latitudes less skin pigmentation allows more penetration of the weaker ultraviolet rays to make sufficient vitamin D while still protecting the folic acid.

Humans adapt to their environment with the same few simple processes we have seen bacteria using—mutation, fusion/ recombination and selection—that occur during the reproduction process only and are repeated during a thousand generations. However, there are critical differences that we must take into account.

> Humans do not reproduce as fast as bacteria do.
>
> On average, humans have one generation every
> 15 to 20 years. One thousand human generations
> take about 15,000 to 20,000 years.
>
> Human adaptation to environmental change
> is time consuming.

The Hottentots have been living in southern Africa for several thousand years. Their skin pigmentation is lighter than the skin pigmentation of the Zulus living in the same area. The Zulus came from lower latitudes closer to the tropics about 1,000 years ago. For the transplanted Zulus 1,000 years (± 60 generations) in their new habitat have not sufficed to alter the pigmentation of their skin.

As a consequence of the time humans need to adapt to UV radiation, people from tropical regions migrating to higher latitudes need to compensate for their original reduced UV absorption by oral vitamin D supplementation. Conversely, people from higher latitudes exposing their lighter skin to the stronger ultraviolet radiation of the tropics need to compensate for the effect of the stronger UV rays by supplementing their diet with folic acid.

What Does this Mean for Human Adaptation to Changes in Diet?

Given what we know about the pace at which humans adapt to environmental change, what are the implications for our adaptability to changes in our environment via our diet?

There are three key implications.

We are still adapted to the diet that was prevalent some 15,000 to 20,000 years ago.

One may expect some partial adaptation to the changes in the human diet resulting from the progressive development of agriculture over the last 10,000 years.

There can be no adaptation to the more recent changes in the diet that have occurred over the last two hundred years. There simply has not been enough time.

Changes In The Human Diet

The Paleolithic Diet

It is widely accepted that Paleolithic humans were hunter-gatherers. They ate what they could capture and find. Paleolithic humans were omnivorous. Some authorities still contest the scientific evidence, pretending Paleolithic humans were mainly vegetarians.[5] However, coherent evidence from a variety of sources suggests that both Paleolithic and Neolithic humans were omnivorous and the evidence Paleolithic humans were omnivorous is from various origins. Here are several examples of that evidence.

1. Skeletal remains from humans living 120,000 years ago and before has been found together with animal bones that are smashed and bear traces of stone tool use.[6]

2. Other evidence comes from the isotopic analyses of Paleolithic hominid tissue, from reductions in hominid

gut size, from the low activity levels of certain enzymes, and from optimal foraging data. All point toward a long history of meat-based diets in our species.[7]

3. Stable isotope analysis of upper Paleolithic humans and fauna from sites in the United Kingdom indicate a diet high in animal protein.[8]

4. The analysis of 9,000 rabbit bones recovered from a cave in central Portugal indicates that the Upper Paleolithic humans who used that cave were predominantly meat eaters.[9]

5. Remains of molluscan foods in the uppermost Pleistocene and Holocene sediments in Spain point toward a shellfish diet.[10]

6. Big game extinction probably led to increased reliance on wild plant foods, a precursor to agriculture.[11]

The Paleolithic diet is the diet we evolved on and for which our genetic profile was programmed. Information from archaeological findings and studies from modern day hunter-gatherers suggest that the Paleolithic diet, as compared to our modern day diet, is characterized by no sugar intake, more green leafy vegetables and fruits providing a variety of carbohydrates, more minerals, fewer omega-6 and more omega-3 essential fatty acids.

The Emergence Of Agriculture

One may expect some partial adaptation
to the changes in the human diet resulting from
the progressive development of agriculture
over the last 10,000 years.

Agriculture emerged some 10,000 to 12,000 years ago.[12] It was a very gradual process spread over thousands of years. The gradual development of agriculture is well documented in the Americas (Table 2).

Elapsed Years	Occurrence
15,000	First hunter-gatherers in America
10,000	Potatoes and other plants in south America
9,000	Corn, beans, and squash displace native plants
7,000	Mississippi plain cultivation
3,000	Speciation of cultivated plants
1,700	Corn appears in north America
800	Corn, beans, and squash displace native plants

Table 2. Chronology of Agriculture in the Americas.[13]

Although historians disagree upon what may have triggered the domestication of plants and animals, there is a consensus that the emergence of agriculture has had a major impact on human diet.

New Food Sources

Agriculture changed forever the diet of humanity. The changes in diet resulting from agriculture are too recent for human metabolism to have adapted to them completely. Although 10,000 years may seem like an enormous time frame over which the human body has been exposed to the products of agriculture, only a partial adaptation of the human metabolism can be expected, especially to the grains such as rice, corn and wheat. **These grains are effectively new food sources for humans. They have been exten-**

sively cultivated and hybridized, their nutrient profiles have been heavily modified from the original strains eaten by earlier humans, and they are now consumed as a much higher percentage of the overall diet.

Some human groups, some families, and some individuals may exhibit a greater adaptation than others to a diet rich in grain and grain products. However, the metabolisms of the majority of humans are still not well adapted to them. In the less adapted, the consumption of a grain-based diet produces symptoms of intolerance. These symptoms cover a range from mild and hardly noticeable to severe.

The intolerance to gluten and to other components of grains has no other origin. Intolerance to gluten is one of the most under-diagnosed health conditions. It affects about two million Americans.[14] As we shall see later, intolerance means much more than we have been led to think.

More Recent Changes

There can be no adaptation to the more recent
changes in the diet that have occurred
over the last two hundred years.
There simply has not been enough time.

Further along in this book the reader will find strong arguments supporting the hypothesis that the suffering, the health deterioration and the premature death of many Americans result primarily, if not exclusively, from changes in the diet we have had no time to adapt to. For the time being, suffice it to say that over the last two hundred years large-scale industrial agriculture, food refining and processing, and unlucky diet guidance have changed the American diet, resulting in a profound imbalance between what the American diet contains and the actual nutritional needs of Americans.

The Imbalances of the American Diet

The American diet contains too many carbohydrates in the form of sugar and starch, while other more important carbohydrates are scarce or missing. Of the two essential fatty acids (EFAs) we need, one is abundant in the American diet, while the other is rare or absent. Since fatty acids come in fat, the low-fat obsession of the American diet only exaggerates the discrepancy between the two EFAs. The American diet is also notoriously deficient in minerals and vitamins, and it contains too many additives and too many calories. Altogether we have four excesses and three deficiencies, the seven deadly sins of the American diet (Figure 1).

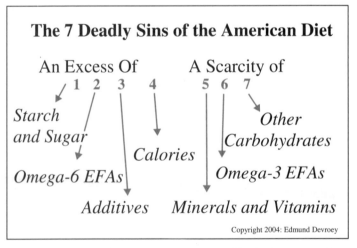

Figure 1. The American diet contains an excess of both glucose and fructose, while other carbohydrates are scarce or absent. Omega-6 essential fatty acids are abundant; the omega-3 essential fatty acids are rare. The diet also contains too many additives and calories and is deficient in minerals and vitamins.

> The combination of these excesses and deficiencies
> contributes to health deterioration in multiple ways.

In this book we shall explore each excess and deficiency of the American diet and analyze its impact on our health. Our exploration will begin with the most deadly sin of them all, the excess of carbohydrates in the form of sugar and starch. But before we look at how they are affecting our health we will want to refresh and review our understanding of carbohydrates.

Chapter 2

Carbohydrates

Summary

In nature carbohydrates exist in plants in a large variety of simple and complex forms.[15] Plants make carbohydrates in large quantity, we cannot. We have to get the carbohydrates we need from our food.

The first disturbing fact about the American diet, in contrast to the Paleolithic diet—the diet we are still adapted to, is that our diet contains way too many carbohydrates in the form of sugars and starches. As we shall see, a dietary excess of sugar and starch is the causal factor of a long list of health disturbances.

The second disturbing fact about our diet is that other carbohydrates that are important in organ structure and cell communication are scarce in the American diet.

What is a Carbohydrate?

The Structure of a Carbohydrate

A carbohydrate is an organic molecule containing atoms of carbon, hydrogen and oxygen. The core of a carbohydrate is made of a string of carbon atoms attached to each other. Atoms attach to each other by the kind of "handles" they have. Atoms come with a different number of handles and some atoms have a variable number of handles. Carbon (Symbol: C), Hydrogen (H) and Oxygen (O) have a fixed number of handles: C has four, O has two, and H has only one (Figure 2).

$$-\overset{\displaystyle |}{\underset{\displaystyle |}{C}}- \quad -O- \quad -H$$

Figure 2. A carbon atom has four handles, oxygen has two, and hydrogen only one.

The oxygen and the hydrogen atoms in a carbohydrate molecule are found in the proportion they occur in a water molecule. (A water molecule is made up of one oxygen and two hydrogen atoms). Hence, in the word "carbohydrate" *carbo* stands for carbon and *hydrate* refers to water. Another term for carbohydrate is the word *saccharide* which means "with a sweet taste." Here is a helpful trick for recognizing carbohydrates. Almost all names of carbohydrates end with the letters *o-s-e*. When you see a word with *ose* at the end, you will automatically know it is a carbohydrate.

The Variety of Carbohydrates

Carbohydrates come in all sizes. Some carbohydrates have only three carbons, others have more. The most common carbohydrates have six or a multiple of six carbon atoms.

Monosaccharides

A carbohydrate with three atoms of carbon is a triose (*tri* = three). A carbohydrate with five carbons is a pentose (*pent* comes from *penta* = five). A carbohydrate with six carbons—the one we will encounter most often—is a hexose (*hex* comes from *hexa* = six). Of these, glucose is the most well known. Together the trioses, pentoses and hexoses form the family of monosaccharides (*mono* = single), the simplest carbohydrate molecules.

ANATOMY OF A MONOSACCHARIDE

The glucose molecule is the prototype of a carbohydrate. It contains six atoms of carbon, six atoms of oxygen and twelve (or eleven) atoms of hydrogen. Glucose is found in sugar (refined or not) and in starch. As it is always helpful to have a visual image to better understand what we are talking about, chemists have provided us with different formulas to illustrate molecules.

THE EMPIRICAL FORMULA

The empirical formula of a molecule only indicates the types of atoms involved and their numbers. Figure 3 presents the empirical formula of a glucose molecule.

$$C_6 \ O_6 \ H_{12}$$

Figure 3. The empirical formula of a glucose molecule indicates the atoms involved and their number only.

The Visual Presentation

In a glucose molecule the carbon atoms are attached to each other in a row forming the spine of the molecule. This is easily seen in more visual presentations of the molecules.[16] Carbohydrates share with almost all molecules of life—fats and proteins included—the characteristic of having a core of carbon atoms. One can truly say that life on earth is organized around a carbon spine.

Disaccharides, Polysaccharides.

More complex carbohydrates are made up of two or more monosaccharides bound together. A carbohydrate made up of only two monosaccharides is a disaccharide (*di* = two). A carbohydrate made up of more than six monosaccharides is a polysaccharide (*poly* = numerous, multiple). Starch is a polysaccharide.

Complex Polysaccharides

Carbohydrates also occur bound to other types of molecules. Carbohydrates bound to proteins are named *glycoproteins* if the combination of the carbohydrates with proteins contains more of the first and are named *proteoglycans* if the resulting molecule contains more proteins than carbohydrates. Later in this book we will encounter glycoproteins that are found in cell membranes and that are essential to cell communication.

Carbohydrates in Nature

A Great Variety of Carbohydrates in Plants

In plants carbohydrates come in a large variety of forms. Some of the carbohydrates found in plants are simple molecules. Others come as much larger molecules formed of sequences of identical units. Starches, for example, are polysaccharides made of sequences or strings of glucose. Still other plant carbohydrates are part of complex molecules that contain a variety of different carbohydrates as well as other molecules such as proteins or lipids.

SIMPLE CARBOHYDRATES

Some of them are simple molecules, quite similar to the

glucose molecule we have just seen, and they contain a limited number of carbon, oxygen and hydrogen atoms. The following list is a small selection of the simple plant carbohydrates whose names you may already be familiar with: cellulose, fructose, inositol, inulin, maltose, mannitol, phytic acid, soluble fiber, sorbitol, sucrose, and xylitol.[17]

MORE ELABORATED SIMPLE CARBOHYDRATES

Many simple carbohydrate molecules carry an appendix. That additional element confers specific properties to the carbohydrate and it becomes part of the name. For example, an atom of nitrogen (N) with two adjacent hydrogen (H) atoms is known as an "amino" group. When an amino group is attached to a carbohydrate the suffix *amine* is added to the name of the participating carbohydrate, e.g., glucosamine. Another appendix found on simple carbohydrates is the "acetyl" group, which is, in fact, the core of a molecule of vinegar (CH3-COOH). An example is N-acetyl glucosamine.

COMPLEX CARBOHYDRATES

Aside from their simple forms, carbohydrates also come in complex molecules. Complex molecules can be formed of successive identical simple carbohydrates. Examples are starch, glycogen and fructans.[18] Complex carbohydrates also come in molecules containing multiples units of more than only one simple carbohydrate. Examples are the arabinoglycans, which are highly branched polysaccharides consisting of galactose and arabinose molecules. Arabinoglycans are found in soya beans.

Other complex carbohydrates are molecules that contain lipids, proteins, fatty acids or amino acids and have such important functions in life that their discovery led to the rise and development of Glucoscience, a whole new section of biochemistry.[19]

Carbohydrates in Food

Few people on this planet are aware of the fact that most of the 195,000 species of flowering plants are edible. Given that fact, it is noteworthy that fewer than 300 of these plant species are used for food. And you may find this next fact to be even more amazing. Today, 7 plant species provide approximately 90% of the food supply of human and domesticated animals in the form of grains—wheat, corn, rice and barley.[20]

The carbohydrates in food are mainly glucose, fructose and galactose. Glucose, fructose and galactose are found in grains, potatoes, sugar and milk. Grain and potato contain glucose in the form of starches. Sugar is sucrose. Sucrose is a molecule of glucose bound to a molecule of fructose. Sucrose comes in vegetables, fruit, sugarcane and beets.

Milk contains lactose. Lactose is made of one molecule of glucose attached to one molecule of galactose (Table 3). In nature, galactose does not exist as a monosaccharide.

Molecule	Family	Components
Glucose	Monosaccharide	Glucose
Fructose	Monosaccharide	Fructose
Sucrose	Disaccharide	Glucose Fructose
Lactose	Disaccharide	Glucose Galactose
Starch	Polysaccharide	Glucose

Table 3. Sucrose contains glucose and fructose. Lactose contains glucose and galactose. Starch contains glucose only.

Glucose, fructose and galactose have very similar chemical formulas. Glucose and galactose possess the same numbers of carbon (6), oxygen (6), and hydrogen (12-11) atoms. However, the three molecules differ by the spatial orientation of the atoms. It gives them slightly different properties.[21]

Glucose

Glucose is abundant in plants under the form of starch. Starch is a polymer (a larger molecule made up of repeating units) of glucose and the storage form of glucose in plants.

Fructose

Fructose occurs in plants under various forms. It occurs as a monosaccharide or it can be bound to a molecule of glucose to form the disaccharide sucrose. (Refined white sugar is sucrose.) Fructose also comes in various complex polysaccharides.

Galactose

In nature, galactose does not occur alone. Instead it is always bound to another molecule. Bound to glucose it forms the disaccharide lactose (milk sugar).

Carbohydrates in Human Biochemistry

History

During hundreds of thousands of years humans and their ancestors have been exposed to the many carbohydrates existing in the fruits, the leaves and the roots of plants they were eating. It is not surprising that eventually several carbohydrates made their way into human biochemistry. Of all these carbohydrates, one—the monosaccharide glucose—became the prevalent carbohydrate in our blood circulation.

> The glucose molecule circulating in our
> blood is exactly the same molecule as the
> glucose molecule found in plants.

Intestinal Absorption

The glucose in our blood comes from the glucose in our diet. The glucose we find in food is readily absorbed in the intestine.

> There is no regulation for the glucose absorption in
> the intestine and there is no limit to that absorption.

Storage Capacity

The glucose we eat and do not use is immediately stored in our cells. The cells most involved in glucose storage are the muscle cells, the cells of the liver and the fat cells (adipocytes). Muscle and liver cells have a limited capacity for the storage of glucose under the form of glycogen. Adipocytes change glucose into fat and their storage of fat is unlimited.

Glucose as Fuel

The belief is widespread that glucose is the principal fuel for our cells and, consequently, that a high carbohydrate diet is best for health and for physical performance. Nothing is farther from the truth. Glucose is not the best fuel our cells can use and that fuel can be stored in small quantities only.

Environmental Pollution

Furthermore, with glucose as fuel, cells pollute their environment. Glucose is like gasoline for an internal combustion engine. An internal combustion engine using gasoline produces water vapor, carbon dioxide and residues of incomplete gasoline combustion—among them, the poisonous gas carbon monoxide. Carbon monoxide and other residues are pollutants. Similarly, a cell consuming glucose produces lactic acid. Lactic acid accumulation induces acidosis that results, among other things, in muscle cramps and "hitting the wall," as athletes call it.

A Better Fuel

A better fuel for cells is fatty acids. For a cell fatty acids are comparable to natural gas for an internal combustion engine. An internal combustion engine running on natural gas produces only water vapor and the innocuous gas carbon dioxide. A cell consuming fatty acids does not harm its environment because it produces only water, that is recycled, and carbon dioxide, the gas that we expel with every exhalation.

Glucose Blood Level Regulation

Recall the surprising fact that there is no regulation—no gatekeeper, so to speak—for the absorption of glucose from the intestine (i.e., what we have eaten) into the blood circulation. However, we do have an internal system designed to maintain a consistent level of blood glucose once it gets into the circulation—a secondary gatekeeper, we might say.

Glucagon and Insulin

This is how it works. A change in the glucose level in the blood triggers a reaction from the pancreas. The pancreas monitors the blood glucose level (among other things). The pancreas gland produces the hormones glucagon and insulin and releases them according to the level of glucose in the blood stream. Glucagon restores a crumbling glucose blood level by releasing glucose stored in the liver. Insulin lowers the blood glucose level by pushing glucose out of the blood stream and into the cells (mainly into the cells of the liver, muscles and fat tissue). Other hormones, such as corticosteroids, growth hormone, androgens, estrogens and thyroid hormone, also influence the level of glucose in circulation although to a much lesser extent.

Therefore in our ancestors (and still in us) moderate fluctuations of the blood glucose level were (and are) corrected by a moderate increase of the glucagon or insulin released by the pancreas. The operative words here are "moderate fluctuations."

The regulatory system that maintains the glucose level in blood circulation within normal range works perfectly, as long as there is no overload of glucose intake.

Chapter 3

An Excess of Starch and Sugar

The Facts

Remembering that the Paleolithic diet is the diet that our bodies are best adapted to, we would do well to consider it the single most important dietary guideline we have. But do we? Today carbohydrates constitute the bulk of the American diet, contributing 60 to 65% of our daily calorie intake. That percentage is much higher than it was in the Paleolithic diet.[22] The significance of this fact is far reaching. Out of balance, our increased carbohydrate consumption is a considerable physiological stress factor in and of itself. Beyond that, the "modern" carbohydrates we eat are essentially foreign to the Paleolithic diet-adapted human body. Let us take a closer look at what has changed and why.

The carbohydrates we eat are primarily in the form of starch and sugar. This high percentage of starch and sugar in the actual American diet is the result of two key historical circumstances.

Agriculture

The first circumstance is the development of agriculture, which started more than 10,000 years ago. As man switched from a hunter-gatherer to an agrarian lifestyle, agriculture became the dominant organizing feature of human community. Food plants came to be cultivated for their reliability, productivity and ability to be stored and transported. Outstanding among these were and are the cereal grains. Thus, the development of agriculture resulted in the prolific production of starch-based carbohydrates and in a significant reduction in the variety of other carbohydrates in the diet.[23] Consider this astonishing change from the Paleolithic diet. The hunter-gatherers forage among thousands of plants and consume all of their edible parts. But when man becomes agrarian now fewer than 300 plants are used in agriculture. Of these, only 7 plants come to provide 90% of human food supply, most of them cereals, i.e., starches. The four most abundant cereals are wheat, maize (corn), rice and barley. Today, starch from grains forms the base of the food recommendations published by the U.S. Department of Agriculture.[24] Starch is digested and broken down into its constituent, glucose—the same glucose as the glucose in our blood. We know we have no gatekeeper to control the absorption of glucose. As a result, the starch-rich American diet is a constant burden for our blood sugar regulatory system that is designed to regulate only moderate fluctuations of the blood sugar level, as we have seen in the previous chapter.

Refined Sugar

The second key circumstance is of more recent occurrence: refined sugar made its debut. Two hundred years ago refined sugar started invading an already starch-rich diet.[25]

Refined sugar is sucrose. Sucrose is made of one molecule of the monosaccharide glucose and one molecule of the monosaccharide fructose. Refined sugar is bad for two reasons. Refined sugar is digested faster than the sugar and starch that comes in fruit and vegetables. As a consequence, the blood sugar level—already maintained at an inappropriately high level by the starch-rich American diet—now presents surges that are larger than the moderate fluctuations our blood sugar regulatory system can handle without damage.

Furthermore, the refining process totally discards the vitamins and minerals that naturally occur in vegetables and fruits and that are required by our bodies to digest sugar. Among them are calcium, chromium, cobalt, copper, magnesium, manganese, vanadium, selenium and zinc.

Perhaps the most astonishing thing about refined sugar is that eating a little leads to eating more and then more. Some authorities have gone so far as to describe refined sugar as "addictive." [26,27]

The statistics about American sugar consumption are eye opening, to say the least. By the early 1980s the consumption of refined sugar in the U.S. already reached around 50 pounds per year for the average adult. The consumption for the average teenager was even more—about 85 pounds per year. Since then the consumption has jumped more than 25 percent. The actual consumption of refined sugar for an average American adult is at least 64 pounds per year. For a teenager it is now more than 100 pounds per year. [28]

A consumption of 64 pounds to 100 pounds of refined sugar per year averages out to a daily use of respectively 80 to 125 grams of sugar—namely, 19 to 30 teaspoons of sugar per day. This is twice more than the (already lax) consumption limits recommended by the U.S. Department of

Agriculture (USDA).[29]

Soft drinks, which contain about nine teaspoons of sugar per 12-ounce can, are a leading contributor to the increased sugar consumption in the U.S., the country with the highest sugar consumption per capita in the world.[30]

Blood Sugar

What happens if we eat a lot of starch and sugar? As we have seen, the American diet is overloaded with carbohydrates, caused specifically by a starch and sugar overload. Recall that starch contains glucose only, and sugar contains glucose and fructose. This means that the carbohydrate overload of the American diet is, for all intents and purposes, an overload of glucose. Now it gets interesting. The sugar in our blood is also glucose. This means that the two molecules— the glucose molecule so overabundant in the American diet and the glucose molecule circulating in our blood—are identical molecules. That sounds like very good news. If our diet is amply providing us with the very molecule that our bodies are so used to, it must be a very good diet indeed! Certainly it can't hurt to add to our system more of what we already have in it, can it?

There are two answers to this question: no and yes. No, it does not hurt from the standpoint that glucose is natural to our bodies. We are used to glucose in the diet and to having and using glucose inside of us. Yes, it does hurt from the standpoint of quantity. The limiting factor is how much glucose the body can handle at any one time. Simply put, the absence of any regulatory system to monitor and control the abundance of the glucose absorption in the intestine exposes us to a glucose surge in the blood circulation each time we eat too much starch or sugar. (Health professionals call that higher-than-normal surge of glucose in the blood circulation "post-prandial hyperglycemia" [*post* = after, *prandial* = eating, *hyper* = higher and *glycemia* = sugar-in-blood] and you will find more about it in the next chapter.)

The American diet exposes all of us to glucose overload in the blood circulation.

We have seen in chapter 2 that the pancreas monitors the glucose level in the blood circulation. This system has been working in humans and in their progenitors for hundreds of thousands of years. It is designed to handle **modest quantities of glucose** entering the blood circulation only, and this system still works exactly this way. In our bodies, just as in our ancestors' bodies, moderate fluctuations of the blood glucose level are (and were) corrected by a moderate increase of the insulin or the glucagon released by the pancreas.

This control system regulates our blood glucose level by removing any excess glucose that is circulating in the blood and storing it in the cells. Here is what it is good at: this system is perfectly adapted to handling moderate surges of the blood glucose level. Here is what it is not good at: it is simply not adapted to respond to high blood glucose surges, and it is totally inadequate to respond to a permanent high glucose level in blood.

Here is the culprit that keeps requiring that it do what it is not good at: the American diet. As we flood our bodies with starches and sugar—cereals, pastas, pastries, sugar, soft drinks, and more—our glucose regulation system is repeatedly overtaxed.

Chapter 4

Hyperglycemia

Hyperglycemia is a glucose traffic jam. Older cities are unable to accommodate today's modern traffic load because they were designed at a time when traffic was very light, consisting of a few ox or horse-drawn wagons. Likewise, our bodies were designed to handle small quantities of glucose only. Allowing the glucose load of the American diet to enter our bodies results in hyperglycemia—a glucose traffic jam.

The hyperglycemia seen in diabetes is an extreme case of glucose traffic jam. Although diabetes has been recognized and treated for centuries, until the last 35 years it was considered something of a mysterious condition. With the blossoming of genetic research, faulty family genes came to be seen as the root cause of diabetes. Recently, however, the controversy surrounding diabetes has again become pronounced. The long-held concepts about diabetes, taught by national diabetes associations as if they were the "bible," are being questioned once again because the scientific research now clearly demonstrate that hyperglycemia and hyperinsulinemia exist in the human body long before diabetes appears. We will take up this discussion in the following chapters.

But for now we must place our focus where it really belongs. Hyperglycemia is a culprit of enormous proportions and of great interest. Why? Because of the damage it causes and because it is easily preventable. The primary cause of hyperglycemia is the ingestion of too much sugar and starch.

Damage by Hyperglycemia

Glycation

Our bodies can utilize the carbohydrates we eat as fuel even if they are not the best fuel for our cells, as we have seen in chapter 2. What is less known is that via an amazing array of biochemical processes our bodies also utilize carbohydrates as building blocks to create the complex molecules that we need. The production of these complex molecules containing carbohydrates is a precise enzymatic process. When enzymes attach carbohydrates to another molecule, they attach the carbohydrate only at a specific site of the molecule. In contrast, carbohydrates can also haphazardly attach to any of several sites along any available molecule. The random attachment of a carbohydrate to other molecules is termed *glycation* or *glycosylation*. It happens most with the most abundant carbohydrates—glucose and fructose. Glycation is as detrimental to molecules as is the more well-known process of oxidation by free radicals. Both processes degrade the molecules' integrity. Figure 4 illustrates the similarity.

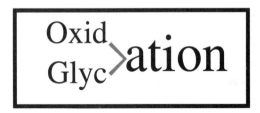

Figure 4. Oxidation and glycation cause the same damage.

Glycation triggers a cascade of chemical reactions that culminate in the formation, and eventual accumulation, of irreversible cross-links. Molecules linked by random carbohydrate links lose their mobility and their function.

The glycation process occurs in two stages. The first stage is the non-enzymatic addition of glucose to proteins forming what are called *Amadori products*. This stage is reversible.

The second stage is irreversible. The second stage occurs when a glucose/protein combination is subject to complex chemical steps involving dehydration, oxidation and other reactions resulting in the formation of Advanced Glycation End Products (AGEs).[31]

Glycation occurs all the time at a low rate. However, glycation occurs at a much higher rate when hyperglycemia is present. Glycation can happen to any molecule.

When glycation happens to a molecule with a high turnover rate, the damage is temporary because the molecule is destroyed rather than repaired, and a new one may replace it. But when glycation occurs to a molecule with a low turnover rate, the resultant damage to cell and organ function lasts longer and becomes permanent for those molecules that are not replaced. Glycation of molecules with a slow turnover is a factor in senescence—the aging of cells, tissue and organs at a faster pace than expected for the age of the person.

Glycated molecules are out of business.

Inflammation

Glycated molecules become trash and attract scavenger cells. This initiates an inflammatory process to eliminate the damaged and useless molecules. Glycation and the resulting inflammation occur throughout the body. No organ or cell is exempt from this process. Most importantly, glycation and the inflammation it causes occur first in the cells that are most exposed to hyperglycemia—namely, the cells in the blood circulation and the cells lining the blood vessels.

Damage to Red Blood Cells

Red blood cells exposed to hyperglycemia have their hemoglobin altered by glycation (*Hb A1c*). Hb A1c is an irreversible stable product. Hb A1c is formed at rates that increase with increasing plasma glucose and fructose levels. The function of hemoglobin in red blood cells is to carry oxygen to the other cells of the body and to remove carbon dioxide from the cells and carry it to the lungs. Glycated hemoglobin is a poor performer. It carries less oxygen in and less carbon dioxide out. Glycated hemoglobin is wasted hemoglobin. The tissue and organs of people with high levels of glycated hemoglobin are doubly compromised because they lack oxygen **and** accumulate carbon dioxide—the oxygen hemoglobin brings to the cells and the carbon dioxide it takes away.

The level of Hb A1c can be measured by laboratory testing. There is a positive correlation between the glucose level in circulating blood and the level of glycation of the red blood cells.[32] The Hb Ac1 level is considered a reliable evaluation of what the average blood sugar level was over the past 3 months. A Hb A1c positive test is not a specific test for diagnosing diabetes. Hb A1c tests positive in all people with high levels of glucose or fructose in circulation, not only in people with diabetes.

Damage to White Blood Cells

Several experiments demonstrate the deleterious effect of hyperglycemia on the number and the function of circulating white blood cells.[33] Hyperglycemia disrupts the communications of white blood, reducing their functions.[34,35,36] We have seen that glycation—induced by hyperglycemia—triggers inflammation by attracting scavenger cells. Hyperglycemia contributes further to inflammation by stimulating the production of pro-inflammatory prostaglandins, active agents in the progressive development of heart disease, diabetes and obesity.[37]

Damage to the Cells Lining The Blood Vessels

An adult human body contains tens of thousands of miles of blood vessels, and the inside of all these blood vessels, arteries, veins and capillaries is covered by a layer of cells known as the endothelium (*endo* = inner, and *thelium* = cover).

With thousands of miles of blood vessels it should not come as a surprise that the total surface of the inner layer of our blood vessels equals the surface of about ten tennis courts. Should you wrap together the inner layer of all your blood vessels, the wrapped volume would equal the volume of the liver, the largest of all human organs. **This is to say that the inner layer of our blood vessels itself is a major organ in the body.**

One may think of this cell layer as a Teflon coating. The function of the cells of the endothelium is to facilitate the blood flow by opposing (like a Teflon coating) the sticking of blood particles and blood cells to the wall of the blood vessels.

There are several explanations for the damage caused by hyperglycemia to the cells lining the blood vessels. They all boil down to the fact that hyperglycemia causes endothelial cells to produce free radicals that initiate and maintain inflammation.[38,39] Free radical production increases the adhesion of lymphocytes to the cells lining the blood vessels,[40] which is the initial step toward plaque build up. Plaque progressively narrows the arteries with all the consequences of a reduced blood flow.[41] The blood flow to an organ is its sole lifeline. The blood flow supplies oxygen and nutrients while carrying away waste products Reduced blood flow is the underlying cause of heart attacks and stroke, among other ailments. Disease strikes when the impact of decreased oxygen supply and insufficient waste removal reaches the breaking point. Plaque does not occur overnight. It is a very slow process that takes decades before it reaches dangerous proportions.

Plaque occurs most frequently in the areas where mechanical stress is stronger and adds its effect to the damage caused by hyperglycemia. Mechanical stress is stronger in the large arteries, the coronary arteries and in the arteries of the legs. The large arteries close to the heart and the coronary arteries are subject to greater blood pressure because of their vicinity to the heart itself, and the arteries in the legs are subject to the hydrostatic pressure of the leg-to-thorax blood column. The heightened pressure in those locations translates into increased mechanical stress to those arteries.

The Obsolete Cholesterol Hypothesis

The "Cholesterol Hypothesis" was based on the years-old speculation by scientists that high cholesterol in humans was caused by our eating foods high in cholesterol and saturated fat. There are three important facts for us to know about the Cholesterol Hypothesis: (1) It was never more than a hypothesis based on speculation. (2) It first appeared in

1956 and was rapidly accepted by the medical community because so many Americans were suffering from heart and coronary artery disease that doctors had to start "doing something about it." (We can only speculate on how many millions upon millions of times doctors have told their patients they have to lower their cholesterol intake.) After years of never receiving the anticipated results of significantly lowered cholesterol in humans, scientific research disproved the Cholesterol Hypothesis. It had already been refuted as early as 1964 but nobody wanted to listen to the whistle blowers such as Dr. De Bakey and others who consistently reported that people with low cholesterol were as likely as people with high cholesterol to have a heart attack.[42]

So let us take a look at what we really do know. Cholesterol does not induce plaque.[43] Cholesterol and calcium appear in plaque just as they appear in all scar tissue. Arterial plaque is a scar tissue. The deposit of calcium in plaque has been known since X-rays were introduced. It is the calcium deposit in plaque that makes plaque visible in X-rays. No one has ever advocated the reduction of calcium intake to avoid or reduce plaque. Meanwhile—in medicine, the media and public opinion—**cholesterol is still erroneously cast in the role of "the arch villain."**

Nerve Damage

Hyperglycemia, glycation and free radical production are the primary factors in peripheral neuropathy. Nerves carry information as a kind of electric current. (Physiologists talk about a depolarization process running alongside the nerve.) Like a power line in touch with other material, nerves need insulation. Insulation of nerves is performed by an envelope of specialized cells surrounding them, the

Schwann cells. Schwann cells, like all cells, are exposed to damage by glycation.[44] The results are short circuit of the nerve impulse and transmission disturbance.

Hormone Deficiency

Hyperglycemia, glycation and free radical production in the endocrine glands result in reduced hormone levels.[45] The effect of hyperglycemia on hormone production and hormone utilization are further addressed in chapter 13 where we discuss calorie excess, overweight and obesity.

Impaired Immune Response

Hyperglycemia, glycation and free radical production contribute to impairment of the immune response and the development of infection.[46] Other diet-related factors disturb immunity and inflammation even more as we shall see in chapter 10, where we consider the effects of the essential fatty acid imbalance of the American diet.

Damage by Fructose

Until recently it was believed that dietary fructose—as opposed to the glucose from starch and from sugar—produces a lesser rise in plasma glucose. Based on that belief, diabetics were encouraged to use fructose.[47] Indeed, the lesser effect of fructose on the blood sugar level has been confirmed by recent investigations. However, these studies have also demonstrated that in healthy volunteers, as well as in people with diabetes, fructose has a higher chemical affinity for proteins than does the glucose molecule. Consequently, the random attachment of fructose to other molecules causes even more damage than the random attachment of glucose.[48] Fructose sticks more than glucose. We shall see in chapters 5 and 6 that glucose increases cholesterol and triglyceride levels and that fructose increases cholesterol and triglyceride levels even more than glucose does.[49]

Chapter 5

Diabetes Revisited:
The Metabolic Syndrome

The Definition of Diabetes

How does an individual become labeled as a diabetic? A person is determined to be a diabetic when glucose is detected in her or his urine (glucosuria). Commonly referred to today simply as diabetes, *Diabetes Mellitus* means "sweet urine." How this old-fashioned name came into being is quite surprising by today's medical standards. Historically, diabetes was diagnosed by taste-testing the patient's urine. If a sweet taste was detected the patient would be diagnosed positive for the condition.[50]

There are two types of diabetes. They are termed type I diabetes and type II diabetes. Table 4 summarizes the similarities and the differences between the two types of diabetes.

Type I diabetes

Type I diabetes is a form of diabetes which has its onset in childhood. It is therefore also referred to as juvenile onset diabetes. In this form of diabetes the pancreas does not produce enough insulin. It is also called insulin-dependent diabetes because the condition improves when insulin is administered.

59

Type II diabetes

Type II diabetes is much more frequent than type I. In contrast to type I diabetes, type II diabetes is termed adult onset diabetes because it mostly appears in adulthood. In type II diabetes the pancreas still secretes insulin—**in fact, it secretes more than in healthy people.** Type II diabetes is also called insulin resistant diabetes.

	Type I diabetes	**Type II diabetes**
Sugar in blood	Too high	Too high
Insulin production	Low or absent	High
Sugar in urine	Present	Present

Table 4 . In type I diabetes as well as in type II the level of glucose in blood circulation is too high (Hyperglycemia) and glucose is present in urine (Glucosuria). The difference between type I diabetes and type II is that in type I diabetes the insulin secretion is deficient. In type II the pancreas produces more insulin than normal (Hyperinsulinemia).

Different Opinions

Classical medical books say the exact cause of type I diabetes is unknown and refer to genetic factors as playing a major role. However, there is solid evidence that the destruction of the beta cells of the pancreas result from an auto-immune process.[51] Diabetic associations and national diabetes agencies agree that hyperglycemia is an essential symptom of both types of diabetes. They, however, express disparate opinions about the origin of type I and type II diabetes. The disagreement persists even to the present day. Table 5 summarizes the opinion of some national diabetes associations.

	ADA	**NIH**	**CDA**	**DUK**
Cause	A mystery		Unknown	
Type I linked to		Auto-immunity		Immunity
Type II linked to	Insulin resistance or deficiency Obesity	Lipid profile Hypertension Insulin resistance Obesity Metabolic Syndrome	Insulin resistance or deficiency	Insulin resistance or deficiency

Table 5. The American Diabetic Association (ADA), the National Institute of Health (NIH), the Canadian Diabetic Association (CDA) and Diabetes United Kingdom (DUK) have different opinions concerning the cause of type I and type II diabetes.

The NIH demonstrates it is better informed than the other entities cited above. Indeed the web site of the NIH acknowledges the existence of Dr. Reaven's "Metabolic Syndrome."

A Pioneer

Medical progress is incremental. Sometimes, however, pioneers make a big leap. Dr. Gerald Reaven is such a pioneer.[52] In his initial 1988 lecture entitled "Role of Insulin Resistance in Human Disease," Dr. Reaven was the first to demonstrate that a condition in people with type II diabetes also exists in many people without diabetes. The condition is the resistance of the cells to insulin-triggered glucose uptake.[53] It took more than a decade for Dr. Reaven to convince physicians that insulin resistance and insulin overproduction are realities and a matter of health concern.

Eventually accepted in medicine, the concept went by many names. By 1999, the World Health Organization (WHO) had chosen a unifying definition for this syndrome. The WHO elected to use the term "metabolic syndrome" rather than the insulin resistance syndrome.[54]

The Metabolic Syndrome

Fifteen years after his first publication, Dr. Reaven fine-tuned his initial observation concerning insulin resistance. In a 2003 publication he demonstrated that a high level of insulin (hyperinsulinism) is detrimental to many organ functions.[55]

Definition

The metabolic syndrome is defined by the existence of at least three out of the five following symptoms:

1. Abdominal obesity
2. Blood pressure reading of 130/85 mm Hg or higher
3. Fasting glucose blood level of 150 milligrams per deciliter or above
4. Serum triglyceride level of 110 milligrams per deciliter or above
5. Serum HDL cholesterol level of 40 milligrams per deciliter or less

1. Abdominal obesity

The genius of Dr. Reavens' contribution was twofold. First, he separated the concept of "abdominal obesity" from the more general concept of obesity. The significance of this distinction becomes evident when we understand one important fact: Excessive body fat deposited in the abdomen has a far greater impact on metabolic alteration than excessive body fat deposited at any other site in the body. Second, Dr. Reavens listed abdominal obesity as the leading symptom of the metabolic syndrome.

Testing for abdominal fat is a quick, easy and non-invasive technique that represents preventive medicine at its finest. It can catch metabolic alteration in its early stages, long before a cascade of degenerative processes occurs. Abdominal fat deposit is evaluated by the waist measurement. Men should have a waist circumference less than 40 inches (102 cm) and women less than 35 inches (89 cm). A waist circumference above 40 inches for men and 35 inches for women indicates a higher than normal fat deposit in the abdomen.

The "at risk" population is comprised of two distinct groups: 1. All overweight and obese people who, by definition, have abdominal obesity; and 2. Individuals who have fat accumulation in the abdomen without being overweight or obese. Clearly, this second group is more likely to "slip under the radar" and go undetected and undiagnosed unless the evaluation of the fat deposit in the abdomen is adopted across the board by health care providers.

2. A blood pressure reading of 130/85 or higher

Hypertension does not imply that you are nervous or tense. A perfectly relaxed person can have hypertension. How do you find out if you have high blood pressure? The only way to know is to have your blood pressure checked! High blood pressure (hypertension) can be very discreet and many people have hypertension for years without knowing it.

According to the American Heart Association (AHA) as many as 50 million Americans age 6 and older have high blood pressure. One out of three people with high blood pressure is unaware of it. Although the role of hyperglycemia is increasingly well documented in hypertension, obesity and cardiovascular disease there is yet not much consideration in medicine for the hyperglycemia and insulin resistance link to high blood pressure.[56, 57, 58, 59, 60, 61] The AHA says that the cause of 90–95 percent of the cases of high blood pressure is unknown. Yet the AHA and the medical profession still advise us to reduce our salt intake. They still promote the FDA sodium guidelines and the *AHA Low-Salt Cookbook*[62] as preventive measures to avoid hypertension. **Salt, however, does not cause hypertension.** Hyperglycemia does. Salt intake becomes detrimental only after the damage caused by hyperglycemia has reduced the kidneys' capacity to filter blood and eliminate waste.

3. A fasting glucose blood level of 150 milligrams per deciliter or above

The blood sugar level test measures how much glucose is actually circulating in your blood.

A drop of blood is put on a reagent strip. A meter then reads the strip and displays the results as a number. Normal results range from 70 to 130 milligrams per deciliter. Results may vary depending on meals, physical activity, and insulin administration (for diabetics) or level of insulin resistance (for people with metabolic syndrome).

A temporary meal-induced hyperglycemia produces fatigue and sleepiness. After a meal, one should feel more energetic. Many people feel sleepy instead. **It happens each**

time a starch and glucose-loaded meal increases your blood sugar level beyond normal range.

Laboratory tests

The oral glucose tolerance test measures how you react to a known amount of glucose. After an overnight fast you drink a solution containing a known amount of glucose. Blood is obtained before and then every 30 to 60 minutes after the glucose intake for up to 3 hours. In the intravenous glucose tolerance test a known amount of glucose is injected over time. The test is useful to measure the surge in blood insulin levels induced by the glucose overload.

4. A serum triglyceride level of 110 milligrams per deciliter or above

A triglyceride is a molecule of fat. A fat molecule contains three fatty acids attached to a glycerol molecule. Hence the *tri* (three) in the name. The levels of triglycerides in the blood stream vary according to age and, to a lesser extent, according to gender (Table 6).

AGE		MALE mg/dL	FEMALE mg/dL
1-6	days	10-170	10-170
1week-5	years	10-120	10-120
6-9	years	28-85	32-120
10-14	years	33-111	39-120
15-19	years	38-143	36-126
20-29	years	20-140	20-140
30-39	years	20-150	20-150
40-49	years	20-160	20-160
>50	years	20-190	20-190

Table 6 . The reference ranges for Triglyceride blood levels vary according to age and gender.

5. A serum HDL cholesterol level of 40 milligrams per deciliter or less

Did you know that we all produce cholesterol? Yes, we make it from scratch. A healthy person synthesizes up to two grams of cholesterol per day. Did you know that an average diet—with no cholesterol restriction—adds only 500 milligrams per day of cholesterol to your own production? Contrary to what many people have been led to believe, cholesterol is not poison nor is it a waste product. It is an essential molecule in human biochemistry.

The story of the cholesterol tests is one of successive adaptation of laboratory investigation to the medical shift of interest. After decades of attention to the total cholesterol level only, medicine now focuses on the complex molecules that carry (among other things) cholesterol in circulating blood. There are different cholesterol carriers. The High Density Lipoproteins (HDL), the Low Density Lipoproteins (LDL), and the Very Low Density Lipoproteins (VLDL). Today much value is attached to the HDL and the LDL levels and to the HDL to LDL ratio.

People with the metabolic syndrome (and people with type II diabetes) commonly have an elevated triglyceride level, normal or slightly elevated LDL-cholesterol levels and low HDL-cholesterol levels.

HDL is referred to as the "good" cholesterol, while LDL is considered the "bad" one. Consequently, a low level of HDL and an elevated level of LDL are considered risk factors. The recommended ranges of HDL cholesterol (Table 7) vary by gender, not by age, while the recommended ranges for LDL (Table 8) and for VLDL (Table 9) vary by age, not by gender.

RISK	MALE mg/dL	FEMALE mg/dL
Average	45	55

Table 7. The risk reference ranges for High Density Lipoproteins vary according to gender.

AGE	mg/dL	RISK
2-19	<110	Desirable
	>125	High
	130-159	Borderline high

Table 8. The risk reference ranges for Low Density Lipoproteins vary according to age.

AGE	mg/dL	RISK
2-19	<170	Desirable
	>185	High
	200-239	Borderline high

Table 9. The risk reference ranges for Very Low Density Lipoproteins vary according to age.

The Latest (and Excessive) Medical Recommendation

Medicine now recommends a LDL level of 70 instead of 110.[63, 64] However, the research leading to that recommendation may be tainted. The authors of the research have ties to drug firms.[65]

The Prevalence of the Metabolic Syndrome

Estimations of the prevalence of the Metabolic Syndrome in the American population vary from 20 to 60 percent.[66, 67] The analysis of the census data from 2000 confirms that approximately 47 million Americans could have the condition.[68]

Chapter 6

Hyperinsulinemia and Insulin Resistance

It is common wisdom that the role of insulin is to lower the level of glucose in the blood circulation. **The common wisdom is absolutely wrong**. Lowering the glucose level in blood is at best a trivial effect of insulin. Insulin was not invented by nature to regulate the level of glucose in our blood. Insulin was invented to store nutrients if they were ingested in greater quantity than what could be used immediately.[69]

Insulin is a Storage Hormone

Insulin causes proteins, fats, minerals and glucose to be stored in varying tissues. Where is the glucose stored? Glucose is stored mainly in the liver, in the muscles and in fat tissue. The glucose storage capacity of the liver is limited. The storage capacity of muscles is very limited. The storage capacity of fat tissue is unlimited. So what do fat cells do with glucose? They make fat from it. Because of this particular condition of the glucose storage, all the glucose that muscle and liver cannot handle becomes fat in fat tissue. The starch and sugar excess in the American diet responsible for hyperglycemia in a large fraction of the population is the leading cause of the obesity epidemic.

Insulin is Not Only a Storage Hormone

Insulin does much more than only storing excess nutrients. Insulin also influences the blood lipids, monitors cell multiplication, influences the production and the utilization of other hormones and modulates gene expression.

Cholesterol and Triglycerides

Insulin, the storage hormone, inhibits the utilization of fat as a source of energy. A low HDL cholesterol and a high plasma triglyceride level are typically seen in people with hyperinsulinemia.[70]

The easiest way to lower elevated cholesterol and triglycerides is to reduce abnormally high insulin secretion by lowering glucose and starch intake.
Medicine has still a long way to go before prescribing such a simple treatment.

Cell Multiplication

The structure of insulin is very similar to a key component of the growth factor molecule.[71] This mimicry allows insulin to somehow activate the cell's growth factor receptors, promoting cell growth and cell multiplication. An example of what can happen is when overweight babies are born to mothers who have "pregnancy diabetes." [72] Another example is the association of hyperinsulinemia with an increased risk of breast cancer and with a poorer survival rate after a breast cancer diagnosis. [73] High insulin levels are also associated with breast hypertrophy and the growth of multiple cysts in breast tissue as well as in other organs. [74,75]

Hormone Disturbances

Several hormone disturbances are found to be associated with hyperglycemia and hyperinsulinemia. Examples are an inability to utilize thyroid hormone and the overproduction of androgens.

THYROID HORMONE

The thyroid gland produces tetraiodothyronine (T4), a pro-hormone that contains 4 atoms of iodine, and triiodothyronine (T3), a more active hormone that contains 3 atoms of iodine only. The thyroid gland produces much more T4 than T3 and releases both in the blood circulation. The liver changes T4 into T3 by removal of one iodine atom. T4 and T3 activate the metabolism of all our cells, including how much food cells use for energy. T3 is 15 times more efficient in activating the cell's metabolism than T4. **Insulin reduces the making of T3 by the liver, reducing the use of food for energy.**

ANDROGENS

Hyperinsulinemia is linked to Polycystic Ovary Syndrome (PCOS), a condition of female infertility that is associated with androgen excess. [76]

Gene Expression

It is not surprising that hyperinsulinemia has such profound effects on health and behavior. Insulin regulates more than 750 genes, up-regulating some and down-regulating others. The genes reacting to insulin are involved in cell communication, energy utilization and immunity.[77] In comparison, thyroid hormone regulates fewer than 400 genes.

Insulin Resistance

Hyperinsulinemia tends to push glucose into the cells beyond the cells' capacity. Cells exposed to glucose overload develop resistance to the hormone insulin by down-regulation of the number and the sensitivity of their insulin receptors.[78]

Skin Markers of Insulin Resistance

Several skin disorders with until now unknown or ill-defined origin have been linked to insulin resistance. They are now considered as "markers" for the condition. Among them are acanthosis nigricans, skin tags, keratosis pilaris, hyperkeratosis palmaris and striae.[79]

ACANTHOSIS NIGRICANS

Acanthosis nigricans is a circumscribed darker part of the skin consisting of a brown-pigmented, velvety harder skin or fine little growths appearing under the armpit and other body folds.[80]

SKIN TAGS

Skin tags are small outgrowths of epidermal and dermal tissue that may be pedunculated (attached by a stalk or stem-like base similar to that of a mushroom), smooth or irregular. They are usually flesh-colored and benign, and they occur most often on the eyelids, neck and in the armpit but may be seen almost anywhere on the skin. Skin tags might be a useful clinical sign to alert clinicians to screen such individuals for the metabolic syndrome.[81,82]

KERATOSIS PILARIS

Keratosis pilaris is characterized by rough bumps on the back and outer sides of the upper arms or anywhere on the skin.[83]

PLANTAR HYPERKERATOSIS

Plantar hyperkeratosis is an overgrowth of the upper layer of the skin occurring at the bottom of the foot.[84]

STRIAE

Striae are stretch marks on the skin with a silvery-white hue.[85]

Conclusion

The metabolic syndrome concept from Dr. Reavens is now fully accepted in research and the number of publications concerning the topic is growing exponentially. In December 2004, a Scirus search with the key words "metabolic syndrome" yielded more than 4,800 journal results and more than 10,000 web results, most of which were published over the last three years.[86]

Meanwhile, "hard-wired" medicine directs none of its attention to the diet-induced phenomena of hyperglycemia and insulin resistance. Medicine does not warn its patients or the public about the existence of the metabolic syndrome and the easily detectable skin markers of hyperinsulinism.

Chapter 7

A Broader
Perspective:
How It All Adds Up

Hard-wired Medicine

Medicine is hard-wired. Once an explanation is found and accepted for a particular symptom or group of symptoms it becomes the rule and is automatically applied across the board. One can only wonder what it will take to modify medicine's dogmatic and conservative approach to the human condition.

While I was organizing the data for this book I received the September 2004 issue of the *Johns Hopkins Medical Letter* "Health After 50" and discovered the article entitled "Prediabetes: What It Is. Why It Matters." That article acknowledges that there is something going on in America besides diabetes. It admits that in 2004 it had become hard to ignore the role of the Metabolic Syndrome of Dr. Reavens (discussed in chapter 5). However, instead of building on the discovery of Dr. Reavens, the article strives to weave his revolutionary understanding back into the time-worn concept of diabetes. For hard-wired medicine, diabetes remains a disease ..."The Disease."

The article presents the Metabolic Syndrome as nothing more than a predisposing condition to diabetes and appropriately christens it "pre-diabetes." This position aligns with the reigning medical dogma. Medicine holds that the consequence of diabetes is health deterioration. It does not accept the concept that health deterioration, in reality, is caused by a pre-existing condition that is present many years before the sugar overflow in the urine warrants the medical diagnosis of "diabetes."

What is the medical advice for people that have what medicine calls "pre-diabetes"? They should take prescribed drugs: Glucophage, Avandia, Actos and, of course, Statins. What should people do who do not (yet) have "pre-diabetes"? Medicine puts them on a future patient waiting list: "they should regularly be tested for the condition."

The article "Prediabetes: What it is. Why It Matters" from Johns Hopkins, a leading medical institution, correctly cites the level of sugar (glucose) in blood circulation as the major criteria used to classify people into one of three groups: "healthy," "pre-diabetic" and "diabetic." **However, they omitted the slightest allusion to a possible link between the quantity of sugar and starch people eat and the quantity of glucose in their blood.**

The Broader Perspective

One does not need to be a rocket scientist to connect the dots and to come up with a broader perspective than the narrow vision of the *Johns Hopkins Medical Letter*.

We have discussed in chapter 3 under "Blood Sugar" that

the starch and sugar excess in our diet exposes Americans to a glucose overload in the blood circulation—postprandial hyperglycemia—each time we eat too much starch or sugar. We have seen in chapter 4 what damage hyperglycemia causes and in chapter 5 that hyperglycemia is also an important symptom of the Metabolic Syndrome and that hyperglycemia also exists in the two types of diabetes. Clearly, when we consider the health effects of the excessive starch and sugar content of the American diet hyperglycemia takes center stage in the four conditions. Table 10 summarizes the similarities and differences of the four conditions.

	Hyperinsulinism Insulin Resistance	Glucosuria	Hyperglycemia
Postprandial Hyperglycemia	No	No	Yes
Metabolic Syndrome	Yes	No	Yes
Type I Diabetes	No	Yes	Yes
Type II Diabetes	Yes	Yes	Yes

Table 10. Hyperglycemia—one of the five distinctive symptoms of the Metabolic Syndrome—also occurs after each excessive sugar and starch intake and is permanently present in type I as well as in type II diabetes. Hyperinsulinemia and insulin resistance occur in type II diabetes and in the Metabolic Syndrome only. Glucosuria is present in the two types of diabetes.

Hyperglycemia Takes Center Stage

Although the current state of our knowledge is not yet definitive, many authorities now agree that hyperglycemia is the primary and central cause of an entire cascade of metabolic alterations. Hyperglycemia triggers an overreaction by the pancreas, significantly increasing the level of circulating insulin. Varying degrees of insulin resistance then occur in many tissues, which triggers more insulin to be released increasing hyperinsulinemia. Hyperglycemia also exaggerates the production of glycated molecules (Advanced Glycation End products or AGEs) as we have seen in chapter 4.

The overproduction of AGEs is a factor in chronic inflammation, vascular damage and senescence. Hyperinsulinemia and insulin resistance are the main causative factors in dyslipidemia, cell proliferation, hormone disturbance and mineral loss and contribute to inflammation, vascular damage and senescence.

Hyperglycemia takes center stage as the primary cause of inflammation and the resulting vascular damage leading to heart attacks, hypertension and stroke. **Hyperglycemia— most likely the first alteration in the series—is the direct consequence of the excessive starch and sugar content of the American diet.**

Obesity and diabetes are side effects. Obesity results from an excess of calories. (Hyperglycemia and hyperinsulinemia are influenced by other hormones as we shall see in a later chapter.)

Diabetes occurs when the damage to the blood vessels in the kidney has sufficiently reduced the capacity of that organ to filter blood. See Figure 5 for a graphic illustration of the above.

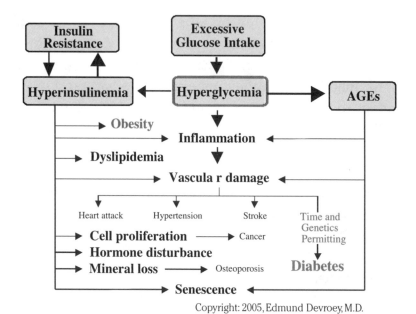

Copyright: 2005, Edmund Devroey, M.D.

Figure 5. Hyperglycemia is at center stage. Hyperglycemia triggers and maintains hyperinsulinemia, and greatly increases the random glycation of molecules forming Advanced Glycation End products (AGEs). Hyperinsulinemia makes cells "insulin resistant," contributing to inflammation and to vascular damage and leading to heart attacks, hypertension and stroke. Hyperinsulinemia and insulin resistance are the main factor in dyslipidemia, cell proliferation, other hormone disturbance, mineral loss and senescence. Obesity and diabetes are secondary events only. Their occurrence is time and genetic configuration dependent.

The Genetic Factor

In any given individual who eats excessive starch and sugar in their diet the extent of the damages caused by hyperglycemia is dependent upon that person's genetic make-up.

If it is true that multiple and widespread genetic configurations are linked to a greater likelihood of hypertension, obesity, heart disease, hypertension and diabetes,[87] it does not mean that the millions of humans with that genetic configuration are plagued by an acquired defect in their genes. The wide spread of those genetic configurations demonstrates that in millions of humans the genes they have inherited from their ancestors have had no time to adapt to the recent appearance of the high starch and refined sugar diet.

> We cannot change our genes. We can change our diet.

Conclusion

Let us review the main points that we have covered in this chapter, keeping in mind their full implications for our nutrition.

1. Starch and refined sugar excess, helped by mineral and vitamin deficiency, result in hyperglycemia.
2. Hyperglycemia causes inflammation and vascular damage.
3. Hyperglycemia triggers an excessive secretion of insulin. Cells become resistant to insulin.
4. Hyperinsulinism is detrimental to health.
5. In many people the condition progresses to diabetes. Contrary to common understanding, however, the diagnosis of diabetes is not the demarcation point for health consequences. Damage to the body starts with hyperglycemia.
6. Time, lifestyle and genetic make-up control the progression of the condition and the extent of the damage.

What You Can Do?

We do not have an automated system monitoring the entry of glucose from the digestive track into the blood circulation. Therefore, we have to compensate by consciously controlling our intake of glucose—before it enters the digestive track.

From a nutritional standpoint we should consider reducing our starch and sugar intake, supplementing our diet with antioxidants, with long chain omega-3 essential fatty acids and with minerals and vitamins. Some herbs may also be useful.

Reducing the Starch and Sugar Intake

Obviously our first strategy is to curb the consumption of starch and refined sugar. It comes as a surprise that some of the associations involved in diabetes management still do not advocate this strategy.

This attitude is in strong contrast with the prevalent opinion about cholesterol. If your blood cholesterol is too high you are strongly advised to avoid cholesterol-rich food.

Why is there no advice to avoid starch and sugar-rich food if your blood sugar is too high?

Reducing starch and sugar intake—the "Low Carbohydrate Diet"—has a long history. One of the first people to promote a low starch and sugar diet was William Banting. One hundred fifty years ago, William Banting wrote his famous "letter on corpulence"[88] in which he advocates a low carbohydrate diet.

More recently, the low carbohydrate diet has resurfaced, in a variety of initiatives. Among them are the Atkins Diet,[89] the "Zone" Diet by Dr. Barry Sears,[90] the Carbohydrate Addict's Diet,[91] and Protein Power[92, 93] to mention only a few.[94] Advocates of the low carbohydrate diet present their programs as the best way to improve health by reducing obesity.

An important recommendation when shifting to a low carbohydrate diet is this: you should reduce your starch and sugar intake gradually to progressively orient your body toward utilizing fat for fuel instead of glucose.[95]

The Glycemic Index of Food

All starches and all sugars are not created equal. Some of them cause the sugar in our blood to rise faster than others do. But how can we differentiate between them? The Glycemic Index (GI) is a solution to this problem. This index is a system of ranking carbohydrates and the foods that contain carbohydrates according to how fast they affect blood sugar levels.

The GI started out years ago as a dietary tool for people with diabetes.[96] The glycemic index expresses the speed at which food increases the level of glucose in our blood. The closer the glycemic index comes to 100 the faster the glucose in the food increases the glucose in our blood. However, measuring the GI of a given food is not a simple task.[97] It is an arduous process involving groups of volunteers that take measured quantities of food and have their glucose blood level monitored during several hours thereafter. The results are then plotted on charts and calculated. The complexity of the process explains why different trials come up with different values for the same foods. Because of this you should consider the glycemic index numbers you may find in specialized publications as approximations only. For more information, see the comprehensive "Revised International Table of Glycemic Index and Glycemic Load" published by David Mendosa.[98] This web site introduces you to more complex data like the Glycemic Load of food which takes into account the percentage of carbohydrates in food. More information is available at the web site of the University of Sydney where most of the work on glycemic index was performed. This web site gives access to a huge database containing the GI of a large variety of foods.[99] In addition, any given food's glycemic index has no absolute value. Several factors alter the original glycemic index of food. The glycemic index of food increases with food processing. Food refining and cooking also increase the glycemic index. Simultaneous consumption of fiber, proteins or fat reduces the value of the glycemic index. The acidification of food also reduces its glycemic index value (Table 11).

Increase the GI	Reduce the GI
Food processing	Fiber
Food refining	Acidity
Cooking	Protein
	Fat

Table 11. Factors influencing the glycemic index of foods

Now the GI concept has been accepted as a way to evaluate carbohydrates for non-diabetic people as well.[100] The high-GI carbohydrates to be avoided include white bread, most cold cereals, potatoes, short-grain white rice and some fruits. Low-GI carbohydrates that are fine to eat include whole grains, brown rice, pastas, legumes, sweet potatoes, oats and some fruits. Reader, take note as you scroll through

Table 12. It may take you by surprise to discover that rice cakes—often thought of as a dieter's best friend—have the highest glycemic index of all the crackers. It may also come as a surprise that rutabaga, potato and parsnip all have a high GI.

Apple, raw	34
Banana, ripe	51
Bread, coarse barley kernel	34
Bread, coarse rye kernel	41
Bread, coarse wheat kernel	52
Bread, white gluten free	80
Cold cereals (average)	73
Parsnip	97
Pear, raw	33
Porridge, raw oats	75
Potato, baked without fat	94
Rice, brown steamed	50
Rice, cake puffed	82
Rice, long grain boiled	56
Rice, white boiled	102
Rutabaga	72
Wheat, crackers	67
White bread, white flour	70

Table 12. Glycemic index of some food. Source University of Sydney

As concern about the carbohydrates in the American diet builds the glycemic index will have increasing implication for the food industry and the way it labels foods.[101] The usual terms such as "complex carbohydrates" and "sugars" have little nutritional or physiological significance and will have to be replaced by others. The WHO/FAO already recommend using the term "total carbohydrate" instead and mentioning the GI.

Aside from reducing our sugar and starch intake—which is the most important step we can take—other steps may help alleviate the damage caused by hyperglycemia and increase our sugar and starch tolerance. All of these steps entail supplementing our diet with appropriate nutrients.

Supplementing the Diet with Antioxidants

Since the damage caused by hyperglycemia is, in essence, damage by free radicals, it makes good sense to supplement the diet with food and supplements containing antioxidants, such as the beta-carotene found in numerous vegetables, and the catechins and epicatechins found most abundantly in green tea.

Supplementing the Diet with Long Chain Omega-3 Essential Fatty Acids

Eating food and taking supplements containing long chain omega-3 essential fatty acids, such as eicosapentaenoic acid (EPA) and docosahexaenoic acid (DHA), reduce the damage caused by hyperglycemia.[102] The importance of essential fatty acids for health, their role in carbohydrate metabolism and the best food sources are discussed in chapters 9 and 10.

Supplementing the Diet With Minerals and Vitamins

To improve our tolerance of sugar and starch we should supplement our diet with minerals and vitamins. Some herbs may also be useful.

Mineral Supplementation

The minerals involved in sugar regulation are magnesium, chromium, selenium, vanadium and zinc.

MAGNESIUM

People with hyperglycemia have lower magnesium levels.[103] The reason is they excrete more magnesium through their kidneys.[104] People with hyperglycemia have less magnesium available to perform the many important metabolic tasks for which it is required. Magnesium helps regulate heart rhythm[105] and blood pressure.[106] Their magnesium deficiency helps explain the prevalence of heart disease and higher blood pressure in people with hyperglycemia. Magnesium deficiency also influences the way calcium is absorbed and stored and may contribute to osteoporosis.[107] The Institute of Medicine of the National Academy of Sciences recommends that magnesium supplementation not exceed 350 mg daily.

The classical signs of magnesium deficiency include heart rhythm disturbance and abnormal muscle contraction and cramps. It is less known that magnesium deficiency also is responsible for confusion, depressive mood and loss of appetite. Magnesium deficiency is frequent in Americans and routinely attributed to decreased food intake and the use of diuretics. **The overwhelming role of the sugar and starch excess in the American diet in triggering magnesium deficiency is always overlooked.**

CHROMIUM

When people with hyperglycemia take supplemental chromium their blood glucose drops. The reason is that chromium is essential for the insulin receptors. A chromium deficiency changes the insulin receptor's affinity for insulin, lowering glucose tolerance and helping maintain hyperglycemia.[108] Chromium in doses of less than 1000 micrograms per day appears to be safe for short-term administration.

SELENIUM

Selenium is a major antioxidant trace element. It is the co-factor of the enzymatic system glutathion peroxidase (Se-GSDHPx). This enzyme system is the main defense line against free radicals. A lower Se-GSDHPx activity is observed in hyperglycemia[109] while we have seen that the damage caused by hyperglycemia is mainly a damage by free radicals.[110,111]

Selenium is a trace element widely and irregularly distributed in the environment. Its availability and content in food may vary significantly depending on the region in which it is grown. The daily requirement for selenium is between 200 and 250 micrograms. Professor G.N. Schrauzer, the world-renowned selenium expert,[112] recommends a daily supplementation of 100 micrograms of selenium for adults taken in the form of selenium methionine.[113]

VANADIUM

Vanadium and its compounds exhibit a wide variety of insulin-like effects.[114] The organic vanadium complexes are 2 to 3 times as potent as inorganic vanadium.[115]

In animal experiments, vanadium is found to reduce hypertension[116] and to have protective effects against cancer.[117] Vanadium in human health is also described as a building material of bones and teeth.[118] **The documented effect of vanadium on hypertension and bone and teeth health may well be related to its equally well-documented insulin-like effect.**

Vanadium is present in a variety of foods we commonly eat. Milk, lobster, vegetable oils, many vegetables, grains and cereals are rich sources of vanadium.

ZINC

Zinc is present everywhere in cell metabolism. Zinc is essential for more than 90 enzymatic reactions in the body. One of these has a direct and positive influence on hyperglycemia. Zinc intervenes in the transport of glucose across cell membranes by enhancing the binding of insulin to its receptors.

Zinc deficiency is one of the most frequent and forgotten mineral deficiencies. Zinc supplementation has been shown to reduce hyperglycemia.[119] The RDA for zinc is 15 milligrams for an adult.

Vitamin Supplementation

The vitamins involved in glucose metabolism are the vitamins from the B group and vitamin E.

THE B VITAMINS

Among the many roles that they play, the B vitamins offer protection to nervous tissue, one of the targets for damage by hyperglycemia.

The vitamins of the B group work as a team. As in a team, they depend upon each other. The deficiency of one results in a reduction in the effectiveness of the others. For example, when that impairment is at the level of absorption, the B vitamin that is less well absorbed may cause a cascade effect in which a third B vitamin is unable to perform its job.

The B group of vitamins include vitamin B1 or thiamin, vitamin B2 or riboflavin, vitamin B3 or niacin (also called niacinamide or nicotinic acid), vitamin B5 or pantothenic acid, vitamin B6 or pyridoxine, folic acid or folate (sometimes called vitamin B9), vitamin B12 or cyanocobalamin, and biotin.[120]

Vitamin E

Vitamin E has important antioxidant properties. It protects fat soluble molecules from destruction by oxidation.

Herbs

Some herbs are said to reduce the digestion of sucrose and as such reduce the absorption of glucose and fructose in the intestine.[121] Although herbs have a long track record in many other cultures there is not much interest and research in our country concerning the way herbs could help supplement our diet.

Chapter 8

Mineral and Vitamin Deficiency

Humans cannot make minerals. We have to get them from our food. Humans and animals as a rule cannot make vitamins but plants can. This rule, however, does have exceptions, and the classification of a compound as a vitamin is species related. Some animals can make vitamin C, and humans can make vitamin D and niacin (vitamin B3). We synthesize niacin from the essential amino acid tryptophan, and we use the ultraviolet radiation of the sun to make vitamin D from cholesterol. The making of vitamin D in human (and animal) skin truly is a photosynthesis process challenging the assumption that only plants can harness solar power for chemical synthesis purpose. In chapter 7 we have seen how significant a role 5 minerals and 2 vitamins play in our handling of glucose. This is a good example of the function of minerals and vitamins in our biochemistry.

We cannot live healthy lives without a continual and sufficient supply of minerals and vitamins. Any deficiency profoundly affects our health and behavior.

Awareness of the Problem

The awareness that a sufficient supply of minerals could be important for health first dawned in the 19th century with the demonstration that some minerals are essential for bacterial growth.[122] These findings were revolutionary. But the actual application of such a concept to human health would have to wait for the future. The context of medical practice of that time was not ready for it.

Today there is increasing public awareness of the importance of minerals and vitamins. The ceaseless efforts of Dr. Joel D. Wallach[123] have greatly contributed to this awareness. In his conferences, Dr. Wallach vividly describes the consequences of mineral and vitamin deficiency and we refer the reader to his books and tapes for more in-depth information.[124]

Health Deterioration

Mineral and vitamin deficiency result in a progressive health alteration.

In stage 1, the body stores are gradually depleted. This can be demonstrated by an estimation of the concentration of the vitamins in different tissues. Urine offers the first telltale laboratory evidence. A reduced urine excretion of a given vitamin is usually seen first, even while the blood level of that vitamin may stay in the normal range.

In stage 2, the blood levels decrease and the concentration of the metabolites diminishes. Stage 1 and stage 2 are not regarded as problematic in healthy persons as long as their supply of and requirements for that vitamin remain constant.

It is in stage 3 that we enter the danger zone. With the decrease in the activity of the enzymes in which the vitamin plays a role, some functional disturbances may be observed, and unspecific symptoms appear, such as general malaise, insomnia, loss of appetite and behavioral changes.

In stage 4 the functional disturbances are obvious, morphological changes are present and they may become irreversible.

In stage 5 the irreversibility increases.

In stage 6 the changes become lethal.[125]

Demonstration

Some people claim there is no benefit to supplementing the American diet with minerals and vitamins. Their claim is based on the postulate that following the Dietary Guidelines for Americans from the United States Department of Agriculture (USDA) will provide us with the minerals and vitamins we need for health. This may have been so at one time but it is no longer the case. Let us demonstrate this by using the same information source, the USDA.

The Depletion of Minerals and Vitamins in Food

Using data published by the USDA we can see that there has been a significant depletion of minerals and vitamins in our food over the last four decades.

Experts Talk

Experts in crop and soil science state that plants require 19 elements. They add that plants will generally die if a soil cannot supply all of those elements. Further, they agree that elements in which a soil is deficient have to be added to that soil to maintain healthy plants.

Fertilizers

Soil depletion is aggravated when plants or crops are taken from the site of production. Under natural circumstances—that is, when plants are not harvested—plants die and decompose where they grow. Their components ultimately return to the soil. Harvesting breaks that natural cycle. Plants draw nutrients from the soil then they are removed as food crops. Of the many minerals taken away in the harvest, conventional fertilizers only replenish three—nitrogen, phosphorus and potassium. And before conventional fertilizers were routinely used, major declines in crop outputs were seen due to soil deficiencies in these three. For example, in Australia between 1870 and 1900 wheat yields declined by 57 percent because of no replenishment of nitrogen or phosphorus.

Commercial fertilizer came on the market about 1900. Commercial fertilizer contains mainly the three elements nitrogen (N), phosphorus (P) and potassium (K) in various formulas. Hence their name, "NPK" fertilizers. Although they have brought relative improvement to depleted soils, the utilization of NPK fertilizers has not solved the underlying problem. Instead, it has created more problems. Crops grown with NPK fertilizers have had lower vitamin and mineral contents than crops grown on unfertilized land. Surrounded by controversy, the value of NPK fertilizers has been the subject of much debate.

Nitrogen (N), phosphorus (P) and potassium (K), among other elements, are essential for the growth and the health of plants. However, the NPK fertilizers contain those three elements only. Plants must find all the other minerals they need in the soil. This is how intensive farming has ultimately depleted the soils. Plants from NPK-fertilized fields may produce record yields, but they lack some important minerals. The plants grown in these fields can apparently thrive without these minerals, but the eaters of those plants—all of us—cannot.

Challenge

I challenge the experts in crop and soil science when they claim there is no evidence that the nutrient content of U.S. crops has changed significantly over time. In complete opposition to this opinion I claim the following:

1. Our food is deficient in minerals and vitamins. If it were not, then why is it mandatory in the U.S. that flour, milk and other products be "enriched" with minerals and vitamins?

2. Mineral supplementation for Americans is vital for us to maintain health.

Demonstration

To demonstrate that our food crops are deprived of minerals and vitamins we will look at the content of two particular nutrients in a variety of food crops—the mineral calcium and the vitamin thiamin, also known as vitamin B1. Two sets of data from the USDA, published 35 years apart, are used. They are taken from *Composition of Food, Agriculture Handbook n· 8* issued in 1963 and *Nutrient Database for Standard Reference, Release 13 replacing SR12* issued in March 1998.

To be able to come to a valid conclusion from the comparison of these two data sets we have to address the fact that laboratory analysis techniques have changed over time—they have improved. It is obvious we first have to quantify a Laboratory Analysis Factor for Calcium (LAF/Ca), and a Laboratory Analysis Factor for vitamin B1 (LAF/B1) that expresses the difference in calcium and in vitamin B1 analysis technology over time. If we then introduce the LAF/Ca and the LAF/B1 into the calculations, we will have a more valid base to quantify the possible effect of Intensive Farming (IF) on the calcium and the vitamin B1 content of food. For our purposes intensive farming is defined as the repetitive cultivation of crops on the same soil with the addition of NPK fertilizers only.

Calcium content per 100 grams edible portion		*a*	*b*	*c*	*d*	*e*
			Raw Data		Corrected by the LAF/Ca factor	
		1963	*1998*	*1998 in % of 1963*	*1963*	*1998 in % of 1963*
1	*Food Grown Without Intensive Farming*					
	Apple	mg	7	7	0		
	Apricot	mg	17	14	-18		
	Brazil nut	mg	186	176	-5		
	Coconut	mg	13	14	8		
	Figs	mg	35	35	0		
	Walnut	mg	99	61	-38		
2	*Laboratory Analysis factor (LAF/Ca)*				**-8.95**		
3	*Food Grown With Intensive Farming*						
	Broccoli	mg	103	48	-53	34	-49
	Cabbage	mg	49	47	-4	45	5
	Collards	mg	250	145	-42	228	-36
	Kale	mg	149	135	-46	227	-40
	Lima Beans	mg	52	34	-35	47	-28
	Squash	mg	28	19	-32	25	-25
	Wheat	mg	36	25	-31	33	-24
4	*Average of the 1998 Results in % of the 1963 Values*				**-34**		
5	*Average of the 1998 Results in % of the Corrected 1963 Values*						**-28.23**

Source: United States Department of Agriculture (USDA). Composition of Food. Agriculture Handbook n°8, 1963, and Nutrient Database for Standard Reference, Release 13 replacing SR12, March 1998.
Copyright: 2004-2005 Edmund Devroey, M.D.

Table 13. Column [a] contains the results of the calcium analysis performed by the USDA in 1963. Column [b] contains the results of the calcium analysis performed by the USDA in 1998. Both sets of results are expressed in milligrams per 100 grams edible portion. Column [c] gives the difference between the data in [a] and the data in [b] expressed as a percentage of the data in [a]. The numbers in column [d] are the results of the 1963 analysis [a] corrected by the LAF/Ca and represent the calcium content of food harvested in 1963, as if it were analyzed with the technology of 1998. Column [e] indicates the differences between the data in [d] and the data in [b] expressed as a percentage of [d].

To quantify the LAF/Ca and the LAF/B1, we first have to compare the 1963 and the 1998 data from food grown without intensive farming. There has been little if any change since 1963 in the culture and the harvesting of apples, apricots, Brazil nuts, coconuts, figs and walnuts. On the other hand broccoli, cabbage, collards, kale, lima beans, squash and wheat have become the products of increasingly intensive farming. Table 13 and Table 14 illustrate our method:

Vitamin B1		*a*	*b*	*c*	*d*	*e*
			Raw Data		*Corrected by the LAF/Ca factor*	
content per 100 grams edible portion		*1963*	*1998*	*1998 in % of 1963*	*1963*	*1998 in % of 1963*
1	*Food Grown Without Intensive Farming*					
	Apple	mg	0.03	0.017	-43		
	Apricot	mg	0.03	0.03	0		
	Brazil nut	mg	0.96	1	4		
	Coconut	mg	0.05	0.066	32		
	Figs	mg	0.06	0.06	0		
	Walnut	mg	0.33	0.57	-83		
2	*Laboratory Analysis factor (LAF/Ca)*				**-14.98**		
3	*Food Grown With Intensive Farming*						
	Broccoli	mg	0.1	0.065	-35	0.085	-24
	Cabbage	mg	0.05	0.05	0	0.043	18
	Collards	mg	0.16	0.054	-66	0.136	-60
	Kale	mg	0.16	0.11	-31	0.136	-19
	Lima Beans	mg	0.24	0.217	-10	0.204	6
	Squash	mg	0.23	0.07	-70	0.196	-64
	Wheat	mg	0.57	0.5	-12	0.484	4
4	*Average of the 1998 Results in % of the 1963 Values*				**-31.89**		
5	*Average of the 1998 Results in % of the Corrected 1963 Values*						**-18.89**

Source: United States Department of Agriculture (USDA). Composition of Food. Agriculture Handbook n°8, 1963, and Nutrient Database for Standard Reference, Release 13 replacing SR12, March 1998.
Copyright: 2004-2005 Edmund Devroey, M.D.

Table 14. Column [a] contains the results of the calcium analysis performed by the USDA in 1963. Column [b] contains the results of the calcium analysis performed by the USDA in 1998. Both sets of results are expressed in milligrams per 100 grams edible portion. Column [c] gives the difference between the data in [a] and the data in [b] expressed as a percentage of the data in [a]. The numbers in column [d] are the results of the 1963 analysis [a] corrected by the LAF/Ca, and represent the content of calcium of food harvested in 1963, as if it were analyzed with the technology of 1998. Column [e] indicates the differences between the data in [d] and the data in [b] expressed in percentage of [d].

Conclusion

The results of these comparisons show that there was a drop of 28.23 percent in the calcium content and a drop of 19.89 percent in the vitamin B1 content of food from 1963 to 1998. Since calcium is of one of the most abundant elements in the earth's crust, elementary logic postulates that the concentration in our food of elements much less abundant in the earth's crust has followed the same trend. Vitamin B1 is part of a group of vitamins that work as a team. As in a team, they depend upon each other. The deficiency of one results in the impairment of the others. The vitamins of the B group are essential for the extraction of energy from food, the maintenance of mineral balances, the transport of oxygen, for brain and nerve function, muscle health and for immunity.

What We Can Do

What can we do to correct for the growing scarcity of minerals and vitamins in the American diet?... Increase our consumption of fresh vegetables and fruit?... Supplement our diet?

Increase Our Food Intake?

To correct for the increasing scarcity of minerals and vitamins in the American diet, we could increase our consumption of mineral- and vitamin-containing food. Because our crops are lower in minerals and vitamins (with about one third less calcium and about one fifth less vitamin B1), we could compensate for that loss by increasing our intake of food by a corresponding amount. An impractical option at best.

Mineral and Vitamin Supplementation

To correct for the growing scarcity of minerals and vitamins in the American diet we have to turn to mineral and vitamin supplementation.

June 19, 2002, the *Journal of The American Medical Association* (*JAMA*) contained a scientific review article by R. H. Fletcher, M.D., M.Sc., and K. M. Fairfield, M.D., Ph.D. It addressed the current debate regarding the use of vitamin supplements and the prevention of chronic disease in adults. After reviewing the body of evidence on this controversial subject, the researchers advised their medical colleagues that the use of vitamin supplements is a prudent intervention in the fight against many chronic degenerative diseases.[126]

The next question is how much is enough?

What We Recommend

We recommend an adult to take two times per day the quantities listed in Table 15. This is more than the RDA and for a good reason. The Recommended Daily Allowances (RDA) are not what we might think. The RDAs do not tell us the amount of a vitamin or mineral that we need to be optimally healthy. Rather, they are a statement of the minimal doses required to prevent the most obvious signs of deficiency.[127] No doubt we are all seeking a higher level of health than mere deficiency prevention!

Vitamin A (as ß-carotene)*	300 mcg	Pantothenic acid	10 mg
Vitamin B1 (Thiamin)	10 mg	Calcium	500 mg
Vitamin B2 (Riboflavin)	10 mg	Chromium	40 mcg
Vitamin B3 (Niacin)	10 mg	Copper	50 mcg
Vitamin B6 (Pyridoxine)	10 mg	Iodine	50 mcg
Vitamin B12 (Cyanocobalamin)	40 mcg	Iron	2 mg
Vitamin C (Ascorbic acid)	300 mg	Magnesium	200 mg
Vitamin D (Calciferol)	50 IU	Manganese	1 mg
Vitamin E (Alpha tocopherol)	80 IU	Molybdenum	100 mcg
Vitamin K (Naphtoquinone)	30 mcg	Potassium	100 mg
Folic acid	250 mcg	Vanadium	100 mcg
Biotin	40 mcg	Selenium	75 mcg
Choline	120 mg	Zinc	8 mg
Inositol	15 mg		

Table 15. Vitamins and minerals: Recommended daily supplementation. (*) There is a lot of confusion about the safe intake of vitamin A. However, 300 micrograms of vitamin A in the form of ß-carotene is a safe dose for daily use.[128]

Chapter 9

Essential Fatty Acids

Introduction

In the preceding chapters we have seen that there is too much sugar and starch in the American diet along with mineral and vitamin deficiencies. As if that were not enough, other diet inadequacies also contribute to the deterioration of American health. They are the following: the scarcity of other carbohydrates than those found in sugar and starch, an excess of calories and of additives and, last but not least, a severe imbalance between the two groups of essential fatty acids (EFAs). Sadly the severity of this EFA imbalance is the direct consequence of well-intended but ill-conceived nutritional advice. Indeed, the advice given to Americans to lower their fat intake has greatly exaggerated the already existing imbalance of EFAs in their diet, with consequences branching so far we are only beginning to decipher their complexity.

Before we discuss the EFAs and their impact on health, let us first have a fresh look at fatty acids.

What Are Fatty Acids?

Fat molecules are containers of fatty acids. Each fat molecule contains three fatty acids. We make our own fat molecules from the fatty acids of the fat we find in food. We also make fat molecules from the fatty acids we make ourselves. This fact is always overlooked as if it were that fat in our body comes exclusively from the fat we eat. We do synthesize fatty acids from building blocks we find in food and we find those building blocks mainly in the carbohydrates we eat. (We will come back to this point later on in this book.)

However, there are some fatty acids we cannot make. As we cannot make them, we must get them from our food. That is why they are termed "essential fatty acids" (EFAs).

You do not have to be a biochemist to understand how a fatty acid is put together.

The Carbon Spine

Fatty acids are composed of chains of carbon atoms. This chain is like a spine. Every carbon atom that forms the spine of a fatty acid molecule supports two hydrogen atoms. The exceptions to this arrangement occur at the ends of the molecule. The carbon at one end of the molecule is linked to three hydrogens. (Biochemists named this the *omega* carbon, after the last letter of the Greek alphabet. Remember this term because it will become important later on in our discussion of the essential fatty acids.) The carbon at the other end of the molecule supports an oxygen atom and an oxygen/hydrogen group, forming a carboxyl group.[129]

The term "fatty" is given to the molecule because the hydrogen coating linked to the carbon spine of the molecule repels water. The word "acid" is added because the carboxyl group at one end of the molecule is acidic. Simple, isn't it?

The Variety of Fatty Acids

Variety in Length and Structure

Fatty acids differ in length and structure. A fatty acid molecule can contain from 2 up to 22 carbon atoms—always an even number. Most of the fatty acids in our food have from 4 to 22 carbon atoms.

The structural differences in fatty acids are determined by the bonds between the carbon atoms. These can be either single or double bonds. A single bond exists between 2 adjacent carbon atoms when each of those carbons is also linked to two hydrogen atoms. We illustrate this bond by showing it as single "handle" that links 2 carbon atoms to each other. A double bond exists between 2 carbon atoms when the handles of the carbon atoms that could be linked to hydrogen atoms clutch each other instead creating a "double bond," a supplementary connection between the two carbon atoms.

Saturated and Unsaturated

A saturated fatty acid has no double bonds between carbons atoms. A saturated fatty acid is a fatty acid with a maximum load of hydrogen atoms. In a saturated fatty acid, all carbon handles that are not holding other carbons are bearing a hydrogen atom. Stearic acid is an example of a saturated fatty acid. Stearic acid is made of an 18-carbon chain.

A fatty acid molecule with one or more double bonds is called an unsaturated fatty acid because it is not "saturated" with hydrogen atoms. An unsaturated fatty acid molecule does not bear all the hydrogens it can. A fatty acid molecule with one double bond is also named a "mono-unsaturated" fatty acid (*mono* means "one").

Oleic acid, like stearic acid, also has 18 carbons. But

oleic acid is a mono-unsaturated fatty acid because it has only one double bond.[130] The structure of oleic acid is exactly the same as stearic acid except for that double bond.

But that one difference—however miniscule it may seem to us—is enough to change both the physical and the biochemical properties of that 18-carbon fatty acid.

Polyunsaturated

A fatty acid can have more than one double bond. A fatty acid molecule with two or more double bonds is called a "polyunsaturated" fatty acid (*poly* means "numerous"). Some fatty acids have up to six double bonds in their molecule.

Saturated fatty acids are solid at room temperature; unsaturated fatty acids are liquid.

Trans Fatty Acids

In the usual unsaturated fatty acid, the missing carbons are on the same side of the molecule. Such a disposition is called a *cis* configuration (the drawing on the left in Figure 6). If the missing hydrogens are on opposite sides of the molecule the configuration is said to be *trans*. Trans fatty acids (TFAs) are unsaturated fatty acids with a twist instead of a bend. Trans fatty acids occur naturally in food in small quantities. However, they are numerous in processed oils. Trans fatty acids are produced commercially in large quantities when unsaturated vegetable oils are hydrogenated. Hydrogenation is achieved by heating the oils in the presence of metal catalysts and hydrogen. This changes the oils from liquids into solids. Margarine and shortening are created via hydrogenation.

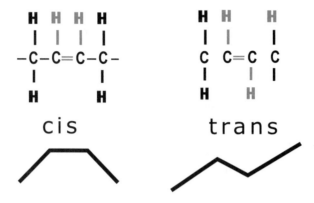

Figure 6. In the "cis" configuration the repelling action of the hydrogen atoms bends the molecule twice in the same direction. In the "trans" configuration, a double bending in opposite directions gives the molecule a "Z" twist

Hydrogenation destroys the double bonds in the unsaturated fatty acids and increases the product's resistance to oxidation, thereby extending the shelf life of the product.[131] Trans fatty acids are also created by deep fat frying. Giving that special deep-fat fried "twist" to the flavor and texture of our foods (think donuts and French fries), we are also giving them a different and dangerous kind of twist. The twist in the trans fatty acids we eat may be a lot more than we bargained for. Whether created by hydrogenation or deep fat frying, trans fatty acids are good news for the food industry but not so for the food consumer. Here's why.

Trans fatty acids are foreign chemicals in our bodies. Put very simply, our bodies do not know how to use them so they accumulate and create havoc.[132]

The problem with trans fatty acids is they do not fit in our biochemistry. Our bodies do not know how to break them down or use them.

Recall that trans fatty acids occur in nature in small amounts and in much higher amounts in manufactured foods. We can see this by comparing the trans fatty acid content of the natural products whole milk and yogurt with the trans fatty acid content of the industrial product margarine (Table 16).

Product	Saturated Fatty Acids	Monounsaturated Fatty Acids	Polyunsaturated Fatty Acids	Trans Fatty Fatty Acids
Whole Milk	2.08	0.85	0.14	**0.9**
Yogurt	0.95	0.35	0.06	**0.03**
Margarine	18	44.89	13.01	**24.1**

Table 16. Percentages of fatty acids and trans fatty acids in natural foods and manufactured foods.

Fatty Acids in Human Biochemistry

As we take a look at the biochemistry of fats, simply remember that "oil" is synonymous with "fat." An oil is a fat. The only difference is that oil is liquid at room temperature whereas fat is not.

The Fat Molecule

All fat molecules are built from the same template. The template of a fat molecule has three long pieces attached to a short central piece. The three longer pieces—fatty acids—extend in space from the central piece much like spokes of a wheel. In Figure 7, the three long pieces are presented as if they were parallel to each other. The 3 long pieces are fatty acids which can be identical to or different from one another, explaining why there is such a large variety of fats.[133]

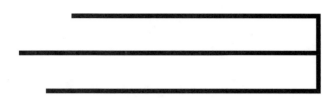

Figure 7. All fat and all oil molecules are made from the same template, a short central element and three longer elements.

Glycerides: Mono, Di and Tri

The central short piece as seen in Figure 7 as a vertical line is known as "glycerol."

A glycerol is composed of three carbon atoms. Glycerol may attach to one, two or three fatty acids (as seen in Figure 7). A "monoglyceride" is a glycerol attached to a single (*mono*) fatty acid molecule, and a "diglyceride" is glycerol bound to two (*di*) fatty acid molecules.

Only when glycerol is attached to three fatty acids as in Figure 7 can it technically be called a fat (or fat molecule). Fats are also called "triglycerides"—meaning that the glycerol it contains is bound to three (*tri*) molecules of fatty acids.

Fatty Acids in Phospholipids

Phospholipids are diglycerides. Phospholipids are made up of a glycerol, two fatty acid molecules and the mineral phosphorus. Phospholipids are essential components of every cell in the body.[134]

Cell Membranes

The membranes of all our cells are made of phospholipids. A cell membrane[135] is a double layer of phospholipids. Phospholipids constitute 65 percent of the cell membrane and all of the cell vesicles, including the mitochondria and the ribosomes where the inner "work" of the cell takes place. Figure 8 is an illustration of the phospholipids in a cell membrane.

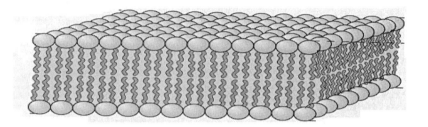

Figure 8. Simplified illustration of the phospholipids from cell membranes. The ovals represent the phosphorus group; the worm-like structures attached two by two to it represent the fatty acids. This illustration is copied from the web page of the Cell Biology Graduate Program courtesy of the University of Texas Medical Branch.

Fatty Acids in Other Structures

Fatty acids occur in a multitude of other structures in the body in addition to fat molecules, cell membranes and functional components within the cell. Fatty acids form an essential component of myelin—the insulation layer around the nerves. Fatty acids contribute to the structure of glucolipids at the surface of the cells that participate in the all-important tasks of cell identification and cell communication. Fatty acids are also a part of lipoproteins. The lipoproteins that have received a great deal of press over the last few years are compounds of proteins, triglycerides, phospholipids and cholesterol. Medicine refers to them to evaluate our cholesterol status: They are the High Density Lipoproteins (HDL), Light Density Lipoproteins (LDL) and Very light Density Lipoproteins (VLD).

The Turnover of Fatty Acids

The fatty acids in our bodies are not static. On the contrary, they are subject to constant turnover. Fat molecules, phospholipids and other fatty acids structures are continuously broken down. New fatty acids are continuously assembled to form fat molecules, phospholipids and other structures. Let us represent this turnover as a carousel.

We Make Fatty Acids . . . from Carbohydrates

The fatty acids from the food we eat enter this carousel. This includes not only the fatty acids that we ingest under the form of fat, but also the fatty acids that we make. Indeed, we make our own fatty acids and we do this very efficiently. We make fatty acids by assembling them from 2-carbon building blocks. But where do these come from? . . . from the carbohydrates in our diet. We make the building blocks for fatty acids mainly from the carbohydrates in our food.

This is important. Why? For the simple reason that the body will turn the excess carbohydrates that we eat into fat. This throws the conventional wisdom right out the window!

Eating fat does not make you fat. Eating excess carbohydrates is what makes you fat. Pig farmers know this very well. They do not feed their pigs fat to fatten them up, they feed them grain. Grain contains starches. Starches are carbohydrates. Food for thought for all of us....

The Essential Fatty Acids

Now that we have some appreciation for the amazing array of fatty acids and the multiple roles they play in the human body, let us get about the business of investigating those essential fatty acids that were mentioned at the beginning of this chapter. They are called "essential" because our bodies cannot make them. We must get these fatty acids from the food we eat.

Two Families

There are two families of EFAs, the omega-3 and omega-6 families. At first, these names may sound a bit mysterious. Let us take a closer look.

The Meaning of Omega-6 and Omega-3

Just as meteorologists give names to the hurricanes they watch and study, biochemists do the same to identify the atoms of their beloved molecules. They give them names. Every carbon atom in a fatty acid is named for a letter of the Greek alphabet. The first carbon—the one that is part of the carboxyl group—is called *alpha,* the first letter of the Greek alphabet. The successive carbons in that fatty acid become *beta, gamma, delta, epsilon,* etc. Then the biochemists realized they had a problem when they looked at the last carbon of the molecule—the only one with three hydrogens attached to it. They wanted to be able to have a consistent name for this last carbon regardless of the length of the fatty acid molecule they would be looking at. (Recall that fatty acids come in many different lengths.) They solved the problem by going all the way to the end of the Greek alphabet and appropriating that letter's name: *omega.*

So what do "omega-6" and "omega-3" mean? Simply this: the first double bond of an EFA occurs on that carbon atom. Omega-3 tells us that the first double bond is found at the third carbon atom by counting up from the omega carbon at the end. Omega-6 tells us that the first double bond is found at the sixth carbon. Mystery solved. It is that simple.

The Omega-6 Family

The prototype fatty acid of the omega-6 family is Linoleic Acid. Also known as LA, it is an 18-carbon fatty acid with two double bonds.[136] In biochemical shorthand you will

see that is written *18:2 n-6,* where the "6" represents the location of the first double bond. The omega-6 family includes
Linoleic Acid (LA), Gamma-linoleic Acid (GLA), Dihomogamma-
linoleic acid (DGLA) and Arachidonic Acid (AA).

The Omega-3 Family

The prototype fatty acid for this family is Alpha
Linolenic Acid. Also known as ALA, it is an 18-carbon mole-
cule with three double bonds.[137] In shorthand that is
written *18:3 n-3,* where the final three represents the loca-
tion of the first double bond. The names of the omega-3
EFAs are Linolenic Acid (ALA), Stearidonic acid (SDA),
Eicosapentaenoic Acid (EPA), Docosapentaenoic Acid
(DPH), and Docosahexaenoic Acid (DHA).[138]

Modification of Essential Fatty Acids

Although we cannot make EFAs, our biochemistry can
alter them once they are in our systems. EFAs are altered in
the same way as the other fatty acids: through the action of
enzymes. These enzymes have pretty fancy names—"desaturase" and "elongase"—but they live up to them. The work
they do is amazing. The body's ability to manipulate fatty
acids via these enzymes is critical to life and health because
fatty acids are required in so many structures and functional
roles throughout the body.

The Role of Essential Fatty Acids

The presence of EFAs in our cell membranes is a fundamental condition of cell health and performance. It is also
from the EFAs stored in the membranes that cells make messenger molecules.

EFAs in the Membranes of our Cells

When we talk about the cell membrane we are not just referring to an outer layer that serves as a boundary. It is much more than that. Cell membranes are not like plastic wrap, insulating cells from their surroundings. Rather, cell membranes are the communication media between cells and their surroundings. Everything that enters or exits a cell has to cross the membrane. Embedded in the double fatty acid layer that constitutes the membrane are numerous molecules, each of which has a highly specific role. Proteins act as filters or pumps for molecules entering or exiting the cell, glucoproteins serve for the reception of messenger molecules and for the identification of the cell, and groups of cholesterol molecules maintain the membrane's fluidity.[139]

There are areas of each cell's membrane that behave like "Pac men." (Do you remember that early computer video game that became so popular?) These develop little bags that engulf exterior molecules that approach from the outside of the cell. These Pac men then carry them deep into the cell (endocytosis). Other little bags or Pac men continuously pop up from deep within the cell and release their content when they reach the surface of the cell (exocytosis), incorporating their own membrane in the cell membrane while releasing their content in the medium surrounding the cell. The quality of a cell's life and its capacity to fulfill its function closely depends on the quality of its membrane. But on what does the quality of a cell membrane depend? On the variety of EFAs that it contains.

Like all other fatty acids, EFAs are subject to intense turnover. It is essential that there be a consistent and uncompromised supply of them, and we must turn to our diet for that.

EFAs and Cell Communicatiom

In any organization, communication between the components is paramount for efficiency. The human body is a very large organization. Hundreds of billions of cells are its individual components.[140]

Blood contains red blood cells and white blood cells. White blood cells and red blood cells are circulating cells. Most other cells do not circulate. They stay where they are and constitute our organs and tissue. Cells are small. The size of a human cell averages 5 to 10 microns in diameter. A micron is one thousandth of a millimeter. If you line up red blood cells you will need 200 per millimeter and more than 5,000 to cover one inch. Have you ever wondered what maintains the unity of the huge number of cells in our bodies? How do they all work together? Cells cooperate with each other by communicating with each other all the time.

Cells talk to each other all the time. Cells also listen to each other all the time. In fact, you might say that cells are like teenagers—very receptive to what their peers, the other cells around them, may say.

Cells do not talk to each other like we do. Cells communicate by producing and releasing chemical messengers. And guess what? Long chain EFAs are the sole raw material for the production of the messenger molecules.

The Making of A Messenger Molecule from an EFA

To make a messenger molecule, cells take a long chain EFA and fold it in two making a kind of hairpin of it (Figure 9). A long chain EFA, as such, has no significance. The folding in two of the long chain EFA (plus some other internal alteration of the molecule) makes it a messenger molecule, a molecule with a significance.

Essential Fatty Acid

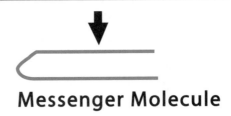

Messenger Molecule

Figure 9. The folding of an essential fatty acid (and some internal alteration) makes a messenger molecule of it.

Prostaglandins

The messenger molecules made from EFAs are prostaglandins.

Two Categories of Prostaglandins

There are two categories of prostaglandins and they keep each other in balance. The prostaglandins from the first category are made only from the omega-6 long chain fatty acids. These prostaglandins increase cell activity. The prostaglandins in the second category reduce cell activity. They are made exclusively from the omega-3 long chain fatty acids. Eicosapentaenoic acid is one of them. As much of a mouthful as that name is, do you find it at all familiar? Yes, eicosapentaenoic acid is also known as EPA and it is one of the active agents in fish oil.

The balance between the two types of prostaglandins maintains our biochemistry within healthy limits.

The Opposed Roles of Prostaglandins

The prostaglandins of the first category increase blood coagulation, a very useful process if you cut your finger. The

prostaglandins of the first category also stimulate inflammatory processes, again very useful when needed. In fact, this
group initiates and maintains immune reactions.

The prostaglandins of the second category, balancing
the effect of the first group, improve blood fluidity, reduce
inflammation and slow down the immune response.

Prostaglandins have a short lifespan. They are made by a
cell, sent out, reach another cell, deliver their messages and
are destroyed.

Essential Fatty Acids in the Diet

Now let us take a good look at where the American diet
stands as a source of the essential fatty acids. Our diet contains more omega-6 than omega-3 EFAs. In the American diet
the ratio of the omega-6s to omega-3s is around 12 to 1. That
is to say that our diet gives us about 12 times more omega-6
than omega-3 EFAs.[141] The situation is worse in Australia. In
Australia the omega-6 EFAs to omega-3 EFAs ratio of the diet
is 18 to 1. Was it always like that?

> In science it happens all the time that the
> truth of yesterday is the error of today.

Do you remember when shortening and butter became
the "bad guys" of American food and cooking? The emphasis
was set overnight on the low saturated fat diet, because scientists came up with a link between saturated fats and heart
diseases. The response from the food industry was swift.
Almost overnight food manufacturers introduced a great

variety of unsaturated oils, margarine and other spreads onto the market to replace the "unhealthy" butters and other saturated fat products. "Unsaturated" became the new buzz word as these oils appeared in processed foods and baked goods.

Nobody realized at that time that
the move resulted in a large increase of the
omega-6 EFAs in the diet of Americans,
tossing the omega-6 to omega-3 ratio out of balance.

Chapter 10

An Excess of Omega-6 EFAs and Deficiency of Omega-3 EFAs

Awareness of a Problem

Many people consider fats to be "the enemy." We look unfavorably upon fats and fatty acids because our understanding of them is skewed in favor of all that is "bad" about them. The list of "sins" that we attribute to fats goes like this: (1) every gram of fat contains more than twice the number of calories of a gram of carbohydrate—therefore fats make us fat; (2) fats clog our arteries; (3) fats are responsible for much of the deterioration in our health. Not surprisingly, these allegations have led to the tremendous popularity of and hype around the low-fat diet.

The Low Fat Hype

The low fat hype pushes grocery stores to offer more products manipulated by having part or all of the fat they naturally contain removed. As a consumer of whole milk yogurt, I have witnessed the progressive disappearance over time of full fat/whole milk yogurt varieties from the grocery store shelves and their replacement by an increasing number of low fat and fat-free products.

The abundance of low-fat foods on our grocery store shelves tells the story: The low-fat hype still intoxicates the public. Suffice it to say that it is going to take a while to re-educate the American public and to redirect marketing strategies and food choices.

A Shift in Research

It took decades to decipher the complex role that the omega-3 and omega-6 EFAs play in health and disease. The scientific understanding has progressively moved from speculation about the functions of essential fatty acids to solid evidence that they are not only essential nutrients to prevent deficiency but are indeed essential to prevent many diseases. Over time the research has shifted its focus from fat to the essential fatty acids (EFAs).[142]

The emphasis is now on two specific areas: (1) the preventive and curative effect of a healthy balance of the two families of EFAs in the diet, and (2) the great potential of long chain omega-3 EFA supplementation for restoring health and preventing diseases.[143] This understanding will eventually turn everyone away from the low-fat diet and render it obsolete. But this shift will not happen overnight.

A Shift in Nutritional Guidelines

It takes years before breakthroughs in research permeate into the daily practice of health professionals and become available to the public. Exceptions to this rule are the products or procedures that are covered by profitable patents and pushed by the patent holders. Needless to say, there are no patents to be had on nutritional advice or diet modification involving essential fatty acids. Thus the abundant and conclusive research on omega-3 EFAs remains largely unknown and unheeded, while medicine, dietetics and health maintenance organizations go right on promoting the erroneous low fat diet.

However, the good news is that a shift is perceptible at the highest levels. There are four milestones that mark the road of this evolution:

A. Research results

B. A workshop

C. An article from Harvard University

D. A note from the Executive Office of the White House

A. Research Results

The significance of some fatty acids was discovered approximately 70 years ago. Several researchers are credited with this discovery. Among them was Dr. Johanna Budwig. A German biochemist, she was one of the first to link health deterioration to a diet deficient in what she named the "linol acids." Dr. Johanna Budwig went on to promote a flaxseed formula to prevent and to cure many diseases.[144]

B. The Cloister Workshop

The National Institutes of Health (NIH) have started sponsoring conferences on the role of the omega-3 EFAs in health and diseases. A workshop entitled "The Essentiality of and Recommended Dietary Intakes (RDIs) for Omega-6 and Omega-3 Fatty Acids" was held at The Cloister in Bethesda,

Maryland, from April 7 through April 9, 1999. From the CD that comes with this book, you have—courtesy of the NIH—direct access to the videos of the NIH conferences covering the topic.[145]

The Cloister Workshop recommends the daily consumption of the following: 4 to 6.5 grams of the omega-6 EFA linoleic acid (LA) and 2.2 grams of alpha linolenic acid (ALA), 650 milligrams of EPA and DHA, all three omega-3 EFAs. The workshop recommends maintaining the omega-6 to omega-3 ratio in the diet at slightly under 2 to 1. The Cloister Workshop also recommends that pregnant and lactating women take 300 milligrams of docosahexaenoic (DHA) per day.[146] Later in this chapter we shall discuss how to apply the recommendation of the Cloister Workshop.

C. The Harvard Review

The third milestone came three years later in November 2002. The prestigious journal of the American Medical Association, published an article by two professors, Hu and Willett, from the Harvard School of Public Health Department of Nutrition that advocated (among other recommendations) an increased consumption of omega-3 EFAs to reduce the occurrence of heart and vascular diseases (H&VD).[147]

The following quote is taken from the article's conclusion: *Compelling evidence from metabolic studies, prospective cohort studies, and clinical trials in the past several decades indicates that at least 3 dietary strategies are effective in preventing H&VD: substitute non-hydrogenated unsaturated fats for saturated and trans-fats;* **increase consumption of omega-3 fatty acids from fish, fish oil supplements or plant sources** *[emphasis added] and consume a diet high in fruits, vegetables, nuts, and whole grains and low in refined grain products.*

It is worth mentioning that the same article dismisses the very approach used in the low-fat diet. "However, simply lowering the percentage of energy from total fat in the diet is unlikely to improve lipid profile or reduce the incidence of heart and vascular disease."

What made the Hu and Willett article a milestone is the fact that it represented a U-turn in medical teaching because it signals a critical shift. It initiates a paradigm shift by spelling out the causative link between the foods we eat and the diseases we get—with the added impact, by implication, of steering us away from the need for pharmaceutical intervention in disease and toward the pro-active role of diet in maintaining health. In other words, "away" from doctors, drugs and being treated for diseases and "toward" taking personal responsibility for our health by eating knowledgeably and well.

> We are what we eat, drink and breathe.

To prevent or treat a disease it makes sense to correct errors in the diet, to supply our biochemistry with the molecules of nutrients it needs and to avoid consuming the molecules that can harm. It makes more sense to do so than to use pharmaceuticals to try to mask what results from diet excess and deficiency.

D. A "Prompt Letter" from the Office of Management And Budget from the Executive Office of the White House

May 28, 2003, The Office of Management and Budget (OMB) from The Executive Office of the White House published for immediate release "Prompt Letter" 2003-13.[148] A prompt letter is a tool introduced by the Bush Administration. While not forcing agency action, prompt letters alert agencies to issues that the Office of Management and Budget from the Executive Office of the President consider worthy of priority status.[149] The prompt letter of May 28, 2003 urged the Departments of Health and Human Services (HHS) and the Department of Agriculture (USDA) to revise the nation's dietary guidelines to include new information that omega-3 fatty acids may reduce the risk of coronary heart disease (CHD) while trans fatty acids may increase the risk of CHD. "Health researchers have found that Americans can significantly reduce the risk of heart disease with a modest change in their diets. The government should make this life-saving information as widely available as possible," said Dr. John Graham, administrator of the OMB´s Office of Information and Regulatory Affairs. In the letter, the OMB recommends that HHS and USDA modify the Dietary Guidelines and Food Guide Pyramid that are the cornerstones of the government's nutritional information.[150]

The Dietary Guidelines affect the content of more than 25 million school lunches while the out-of-date Food Guide Pyramid appears on many food products, providing consumers an obsolete outline of what to eat each day. What is important to realize here is that the Food Guide Pyramid has not been updated since 1992.

The paper from Harvard University and the OMB document focus on the effect of the omega-3 EFAs deficiency in the American diet on heart and vascular disease. The reasons for this focus are evident. Heart and vascular disease accounts for 53 percent of all deaths in the U.S. annually, and about 62 million people in this country suffer from some form of heart and vascular disease[151]—which equals one out of every five Americans. About 700,000 people died of heart and vascular disease in 2001. That is an average of 1,900 people each day, 80 every hour, more than one death every 35 minutes. The human costs of heart and vascular disease are immeasurable but in dollars alone the cost per year is estimated at $329.2 billion.

Comments

1. The omega-3 EFA deficiency in the American diet results in much more health deterioration than heart and vascular diseases alone.

2. The recommendations to increase the consumption of omega-3 EFAs should come with the advice to reduce the consumption of foods high in omega-6 EFAs.

3. There are more errors in the American diet than omega-3 EFA deficiency only.

The deficiency of omega-3 EFAs in the American diet aggravates the diet's imbalance between omega-6 and omega-3 EFAs and contributes to health deterioration in many ways.

Among them, it exaggerates immune response and increases blood coagulation. This significant impact is most obvious when you look at the plethora of pharmaceutical products that we use to calm down our overactive immune systems: cortisone and anti-inflammatory medications. In the latter category we have the entire army of over-the-counter drugs that are known in the "trade" as the NSAIDs—an obfuscating term if there ever was one! NSAIDs stands for "nonsteroidal anti-inflammatory drugs." Let us get you started off with generic names and then see just how many brands you can name:"acetaminophen, aspirin, ibuprofen"....And to all these immune system calming agents we must often add anticoagulants because of the same omega-3 EFA deficiency.

The omega-3 fatty acid deficiency in the American diet factors into many non-communicable diseases.[152]

Among them we include the following:

1. Heart attacks and strokes

2. Abnormal immune response resulting in:

   a. Allergies

   b. Autoimmune disease

3. Chronic inflammation

4. Behavioral alteration

5. Pregnancy disturbances

1. Heart Attacks and Stroke

It is now well established that people that consume fish or other sources of dietary omega-3 EFAs have fewer cardiovascular problems.[153, 154] The American Medical Association published in 2003 that eating more fish and omega-3 EFAs was associated with reduced risk of stroke for women.[155]

OMEGA-3 LONG CHAIN ESSENTIAL FATTY ACIDS PROTECT THE ARTERIES

We have seen in chapter 4 that the sugar and starch excess in the American diet and the resulting hyperglycemia cause the inflammation of the arteries leading to arteriosclerosis. As if this were not sufficient the omega-6 to omega-3 EFA imbalance in the diet further aggravates the process because the prevalence of the omega-6 EFA expands the course of any inflammation.[156, 157, 158]

OMEGA-3 EFAS STABILIZE THE HEART RHYTHM

The stabilizing effect of omega-3 EFAs on heart rhythm involves the movement of calcium ions (Ca++) as they enter and exit the cell. Ca++ ions enter cells through calcium entry channels embedded in the membrane. The concentration of Ca++ around a cell is about 10,000 times greater than it is in the cell. As a consequence, calcium enters a cell readily as soon as calcium entry channels open. However, the exit of calcium from a cell takes energy. Calcium can only exit a cell if it is pumped out by the calcium exit pumps that work against the pressure of the high concentration of calcium at the outside of the cell. Although the exchange of calcium takes place at a microscopic level, this exchange process is, for us, a life or death matter. It is a drama that is both infinitesimal and essential—and dependent upon the participation of the omega-3 EFAs.

CALCIUM ENTRY

The entry of calcium into the cell activates a cascade of events resulting in increased activity of the cell. In a muscle cell the entry of only a few calcium atoms is sufficient to produce a contraction. In the heart muscle cells, the sequential opening of the calcium entry channels activated by rhythmic nerve impulse maintains the regularity of the heart contraction. It is obvious that such a system remains efficient only if calcium is constantly pumped out of the cell. That is the task of the calcium exit pumps.

CALCIUM EXIT

Here is where omega-3 EFAs make all the difference. The capacity of the calcium pumps depends on the presence of omega-3 EFAs in the cell membrane. If the omega-3 EFAs are missing, the calcium exit pump becomes sluggish. Calcium accumulates in the cell making the entry of more calcium a less efficient trigger. In a heart cell, the contraction may become weak and irregular.

Temporary accumulations of calcium occur all the time. Each time your heart muscle has some overload of work— when emotions are felt, during strenuous exercise or when lung emboli create an obstacle to the blood flow in the lungs.

An accumulation of calcium in the heart muscle cell becomes detrimental only if the calcium pump cannot expel the calcium fast enough to prepare the muscle cell for the next calcium entry and the next contraction.

> This is how emotions, strenuous effort, heart attacks and emboli kill people who eat a low omega-3 EFA diet.

2. Abnormal Immune Response

The immune system is a complicated network of cells and cell components that contribute to defend the body. The immune system reacts to the presence of foreign molecules by creating an army of specialized cells and by producing antibodies. Here is how it works: a process that we call "target recognition" directs the immune response while messenger molecules and other factors modulate the intensity of that immune response. Both aspects of our immune defense system, the target recognition as well as the intensity modulation of its response, are influenced by our diet.

TARGET RECOGNITION

All our cells wear identification molecules that protrude from their membranes. These molecules are the cells' "ID tags." Any cell missing a correct ID tag is considered foreign by the immune system and will be attacked. The cell tags are made of various carbohydrates. The role of nutrition in target recognition is addressed in the next chapter where we discuss the scarcity of some carbohydrates in the American diet.

INTENSITY MODULATION

The messenger molecules (prostaglandin hormones) that modulate the immune response are made of EFAs exclusively. Recall that we make two types of these prostaglandin hormones: type 1 from omega-6 EFAs and type 2 from omega-3 EFAs. Type 1 increases immune response, type 2 reduces it, and an efficient immune response depends on the balance between the two types. This is where the imbalance of the omega-6 to omega-3 EFAs in the diet exaggerates the intensity of the immune response.

a. Allergies

When people have allergies, the intensity of their immune response is exaggerated. If you inhale some pollen the normal reaction of the immune system is to make you sneeze it out. If you get sick from inhaling pollen, as many people do, it is because of an exaggerated immune response. Why do so many Americans have an exaggerated immune response to pollen and to a multitude of other substances? Because of the omega-6 to omega-3 imbalance in their diet.

It is good to have enough omega-6 EFAs to initiate an immune response when we need a defense and we are fortunate to have a more than sufficient supply of omega-6

EFAs in our diet. However, we have seen in chapter 9 that the prostaglandins we make from omega-3 EFAs do the opposite of the prostaglandins made from omega-6 EFAs. They slow down the immune response. What happens to people with an excess of omega-6 and a shortage of omega-3 EFAs in their diet? Whenever their immune system starts a defensive action, it runs without brakes and continues its operation far beyond its target by maintaining the excessive response we call "allergy."

Allergy is the sixth leading cause of chronic disease in the United States. More than 50 million Americans suffer from allergies. In 1996 the Centers for Disease Control estimation of allergy prevalence in the United States was already between 9 and 16 percent. Allergy costs the American health care system $18 billion annually and is on the increase.[159, 160, 161]

The cost in dollars says nothing about the suffering of people with allergy. Have you ever had an allergic reaction? If so, you will certainly remember how uncomfortable—even debilitated—you can feel.

Are you aware that what you have been reading about in this chapter and what you will find further in this book gives you the means to mitigate and even avoid such health-compromising experiences in the future?

ALLERGENS

An allergy is an abnormal reaction of the immune system to a substance that is ordinarily harmless. An ordinarily harmless substance that can cause an allergic reaction is called an "allergen." Allergens are found in food. Nuts and peanuts are examples.

FOOD ALLERGY

Six to seven million Americans suffer from food allergy.[162, 163] The most severe forms come from peanut or tree nut sensitivity.[164] A peanut allergy can even be life threatening, causing an extreme allergic reaction called "anaphylaxis" in some individuals. The widespread allergy to peanuts becomes even more problematic when we recognize that peanuts and peanut oil are often used in restaurant-prepared and pre-packaged foods, requiring those with peanut allergies—and their parents! —to be diligent about asking questions and scrutinizing food labels.

Other food allergies exist. Some people are allergic to shrimp. It is worth mentioning that an allergic reaction to shrimp is always much less severe than the allergic reaction to peanuts. The reason for this difference is very simple. Aside from the allergens it comes with, peanuts contain omega-6 EFAs exclusively, the EFAs that boost immune reaction, while shrimp are rich in long chain omega-3 EFAs that are, as we have seen, the brakes of the immune system.

Some people believe they are allergic to milk and diary product because if they eat something containing it they have diarrhea. This reaction is not an allergic reaction. It is an intolerance to lactose, the form of sugar in milk that they cannot digest. You may recall that we described this in chapter 1 as an example of lack of adaptation to diet alteration.

OTHER ALLERGIES

There are many allergies to substances other than foods. Examples are allergies to latex, drugs, insect venom, mold and mildew, scents and fragrances.[165, 166, 167]

Symptoms of allergy can be mild or severe and may affect the skin, the respiratory tract, the intestine, heart, blood circulation and brain function. Severe symptoms are called "anaphylaxis." Allergic reactions affecting the skin include atopic dermatitis and hives. Atopic dermatitis is one of the most common skin diseases particularly in infants and children. The estimated prevalence in the United States is 9 percent and the prevalence of atopic dermatitis appears to be increasing. Acute urticaria (hives) is common, affecting 10 to 20 percent of the population at some time in their lives.[168]

b. Autoimmune Disease

In allergy the immune response is exaggerated. In autoimmunity the body's reaction is even more extreme. Added to the exaggerated immune response that is seen in allergy, there is also a failure to discriminate between what is self and what is foreign and the exaggerated immune response becomes directed against self. (The prefix *auto* stems from the Greek word for "self"). In autoimmunity the immune response targets the cells, tissues and organs of its own body.

Autoimmunity results in a large variety of overlapping health problems that frequently make their way onto the ever-growing list of chronic diseases. More than 130 clinically distinct autoimmune diseases have been identified and the list continues to grow. Some of the autoimmune diseases are well known, including diabetes type 1, irritable bowel syndrome, lupus, multiple sclerosis, rheumatoid arthritis and juvenile arthritis. Others are less familiar, including Crohn's disease, ulcerative proctitis, Graves' disease, Hashimoto's thyroiditis, mixed connective tissue disease, pemphigus, progressive systemic sclerosis, sarcoidosis, Sjogren's syndrome, temporal arteritis and various skin conditions. Collectively these diseases afflict more than 15 million Americans with women being affected disproportionately. Autoimmune conditions represent a significant physical, emotional and financial burden for the society and particularly for the people suffering from it. Many people with autoimmunity take over-the-counter and prescription drugs on a daily basis to reduce their painful symptoms and to help them get through their day.

The exaggerated and ill-directed immune response in autoimmunity affects people in very different ways. For example, the immune response is directed against the nerves in multiple sclerosis and against the gut in Crohn's disease. In other autoimmune diseases such as lupus, affected tissues and organs may vary among individuals with the same disease. One person with lupus may have affected skin and joints whereas another may have affected skin, kidney and lungs. Ultimately, damage to certain tissues by the immune system may be permanent as with destruction of insulin-producing cells of the pancreas in type 1 diabetes.[169]

There is, however, hope for people affected by an autoimmune condition and this hope stems from the involvement of diet-related factors in the development of all autoimmune conditions. In our view several diet-related factors explain why so many Americans are plagued by one or more autoimmune condition. The first factor is the abnormal omega-6 to omega-3 ratio in their diet. As for allergy, the overwhelming presence of omega-6 EFAs exaggerates any immune response. The second factor is the scarcity of a variety of carbohydrates that are required for the immune system to be able to distinguish between "self" and "other." (You will read more about this in the next chapter.) In addition, the sugar and starch excess of the diet maintains hyperglycemia, a potent and overlooked inflammatory agent aggravating the inflammation present in every autoimmune condition. Importantly, hyperglycemia also reduces the synthesis of anti-inflammatory molecules like the prostaglandins that are derived from the already scarce supply of omega-3 EFAs in the diet. Hyperglycemia also stimulates the production of pro-inflammatory agents, including the pro-inflammatory prostaglandins derived from the overabundant omega-6 EFAs the American diet provides.

More Information about Allergy and Autoimmunity

There is plenty of information available about allergies and the autoimmune diseases, and you will find a few suggestions here about how to access that information on the World Wide Web. But there is one point that you must be aware of first: as a rule, the role of nutrition in treating allergy and autoimmune disease is largely ignored.

Indicative of how widespread allergy and autoimmune disease have become in the American population, there are several web sites for almost every allergic and autoimmune condition. To find them, go to the search engine Google.[170] Entering the name of any specific autoimmune condition in the query box will yield a list of the relevant web sites. You can also access the National Institutes of Health information about autoimmune diseases.[171] As you investigate these web sites, do remember that nutrition plays only a small part, if it plays one at all, in their recommendations.

One of the notable exceptions to that rule is the web site of the Canadian Asthma Prevention Institute (CAPI).[172] People with asthma are well advised to visit this well-organized, updated and very informative web site. Indeed, you are encouraged to explore this web site even if you do not have asthma because of the scope of this web site. Among its offerings, the Canadian Asthma Prevention Institute has launched a significant study called "Researching Asthma and Influence of Nutritional Supplements" (RAINS). The RAINS study is the first web-based, international, prospective study on the influence of nutritional supplements on asthma.[173]

People with asthma are encouraged to participate in the study, and enrollment can be done on line. The researchers at CAPI released the findings of their first retrospective survey on the influence of nutritional supplements on asthma.[174] The survey reported results of a group of diagnosed asthmatics that have used scientifically formulated, potency assured, pharmaceutical grade nutrient supplements for a period ranging from 3 months to 6 years. Two of the most significant results reported were that 91.4% experienced improvement(s) in their asthma symptoms, while 88.1% reduced their medications (72.9% reduced inhaler use). The beneficial "side effects" included a reported increase in energy (87.2%), improvements in other areas of health (95.7%), reduction in existing allergy symptoms (85.9%) and improvements in sleeping patterns (72.3%).

3. Chronic Inflammation

Dolor is Latin for pain, *tumor* is Latin for swelling; *robor* means redness, and *calor* means heat. Those are the four symptoms of an acute inflammatory response. An inflammatory response arises each time we have an injury and each time we have to defend ourselves against chemicals, germs or parasites.

An acute inflammatory response is short lived and can be very intense. Examples are the flu, a pneumonia, diarrhea. A chronic inflammatory response lasts much longer, and it can persist for days, months and even years. A chronic inflammatory response is not always the consequence of an acute response. A chronic inflammatory response can start silently and unobtrusively and then develop insidiously over any length of time.

A special mention is made of the increasing prevalence of chronic sinusitis and bronchitis in adults as well as the staggering number of children with chronic internal ear infection. Physicians prescribe antibiotics and advise people to have their sinuses scraped and the ears of their children adorned with tubes. The role of allergy and autoimmunity in those conditions is regularly overlooked by medicine.

As for allergy and autoimmunity, diet correction and supplementation are clearly the answer. Eating less sugar, starch and omega-6 EFAs and supplementing the diet with omega-3 EFAs, minerals and vitamins are the most efficient and least expensive approaches that the millions of people affected by these ailments can take.

Association

A chronic inflammatory response is seen in many conditions associated with allergy and autoimmunity. In fact, the health conditions in which all three types of immune responses are associated are numerous. It may even be said that the division of symptoms into "allergic," "autoimmune" and "inflammatory" immune responses is an arbitrary and artificial division.

As it is the intention of this author to promote the concept of unification wherever possible, let us consider that such arbitrary division may not, in fact, be useful. What does seem to be gained by this artificial division of symptoms is nothing more than erecting barriers between conditions. What stands to be lost, however, is the very real possibility of these conditions benefiting from the same nutritional approaches. Studies are beginning to show that supplementation with long chain omega-3 EFAs brings about improvement in the chronic inflammatory symptoms in each and every one of these conditions: arteriosclerosis,[175] chronic bronchitis,[176] sinusitis[177], diabetes[178] and obesity,[179] to name only a few. In a recent article, the words "Diabesity" and "Obesitis" are used to emphasize the role of inflammation in two of them, diabetes and obesity.[180]

4. Behavior Alterations

We know that the long chain omega-3 EFAs are important constituents of the membranes of all cells, including brain and nervous tissue cells. Here is one example. The omega-3 EFA docosahexaenoic acid (DHA) is particularly important for the retina and for the brain of humans and other mammals. It has a profound influence on the activity of those cells.[181]

The Brain Needs DHA for Development and Function

DEVELOPMENT

Brain development occurs critically during the last months of pregnancy and during the first months after birth. Researchers in Sweden have found that children born to mothers who had taken supplements containing long chain omega-3 EFAs during pregnancy and lactation scored significantly higher on the Mental Processing Test, a kind of I.Q. test for babies. Mothers who supplement their diet with product rich in docosahexaenoic acid (DHA) during pregnancy and lactation are doing their children a favor in later years.[182]

FUNCTION

Not surprisingly, we are finding that omega-3 EFA deficiency in the diet is a factor in the increasing occurrence of brain dysfunctions. Heading the list of these dysfunctions are depression, Attention Deficit Hyperactivity Disorder (ADHD) and Alzheimer's disease.

DEPRESSION

People with major depression have marked depletions in long chain omega-3 EFAs and particularly in DHA in the membranes of their cells.[183]

ALZHEIMER'S DISEASE

Decreases in DHA in the brain are associated with cognitive decline during aging and with onset of Alzheimer's disease.

ATTENTION DEFICIT HYPERACTIVITY DISORDER (ADHD)

DHA is essential for dopamine metabolism which is found to be defective in ADHD.[184] It is known that Attention Deficit Hyperactivity Disorder comes with some abnormalities in the frontostriatal brain circuitry and with a reduced activation of the dopamine receptors. Those findings explain the benefits of drugs like methylphenidate (Ritalin) and other psychostimulants[185] that increase the level of dopamine in the brain.[186, 187]

There is mounting resistance against the use of Ritalin for ADHD. The reasons are the prevalence of side effects which include nervousness, headache, insomnia, anorexia, and heart problems.[188] In addition, it seems that Ritalin may impair growth.[189]

Food intolerance and food additives have a trigger effect in ADHD. See the web site of the Feingold Association of the

United States for more information.[190]

Children with ADHD should also eat less sugar, less food with a high glycemic index, less food high in omega-6 EFAs. Their diet should be supplemented with minerals and vitamins, with EPA and DHA. Children with ADHD should be checked for possible food and gluten intolerance.

5. Pregnancy Disturbances

> The stage for an ADHD child may have already been set in the womb of the mother.

Omega-3 deficiency in the mother may impair the brain development of the fetus and particularly its frontal cortex. Recent studies have provided evidence that DHA is needed for brain development as well as for the dopamine and serotonin metabolism in the brain.

The fetus, especially during the last trimester of pregnancy, has high requirements for the essential omega-3 fatty acid docosahexaenoic acid (DHA).[191] Why did the Cloister Workshop recommend that pregnant and lactating women take 300 milligram of docosahexaenoic acid (DHA) each day?[192] Because brain growth occurs mainly during the last three months of the pregnancy and during the first months of life. Evidence shows that the consequences for the fetus of a long chain omega-3 EFA deficiency in the mother were aggravated over the last 50 years by infant formulas that lacked DHA and other omega-3 fatty acids.[193]

Not only does omega-3 long chain EFA deficiency during pregnancy have severe consequences for the fetus, it is also a cause of problems for the mother at birth and thereafter.

SLOW CHILDBIRTH

The prostaglandins produced from eicosapentaenoic acid (EPA) are indispensable for the easy opening of the cervix at the end of the pregnancy. Slow opening of the cervix is one of the main indications for a cesarean delivery. During the days preceding birth, prostagladins, produced exclusively from long chain omega-3 EFAs, block the progesterone hormone receptors in the cervix, preparing a smooth and accelerated opening.

Without question, the omega-3 deficiency in the American diet contributes to the dubious honor of the United States having the highest cesarean section rate in the world. This is in strong contrast to the situation in the Netherlands, a country with one of the lowest cesarean section rates. In the Netherlands a prominent folk tale extols the virtues of pregnant women eating one herring each day. Herring is one of the "five-star" cold-water fish that ends up on every recommendation list as a generous source of guess what? Right you are ... omega-3 EFAs!

BABY BLUES

Childbirth, long recognized as a major physical, psychological and social stress in a woman's life, is also an important risk factor in the development of mental illness. Early descriptive studies are supported by several reports documenting a mysterious but evident temporal relationship between psychiatric problems and childbirth. As always, when the cause of a condition is unclear, laundry lists of disparaging predisposing factors are published.[194]

Only recently has the mystery of "the Baby Blues" been unraveled. Postpartum depression is caused by long chain omega-3 EFA deficiency. Women who begin their pregnancies with a low level of stored long chain omega-3 EFAs are further depleted by the growing fetus. What's more, their depleted state becomes worse during breast-feeding.[195] In light of the above, the recommendation of the Cloister Workshop that every pregnant woman should supplement her diet with 300 milligrams of DHA daily makes very good sense.[196]

What You Can Do

Are you aware of the tremendous implication of the foregoing discussion? Simply put, we now have more knowledge to make real improvements in our health. So let us summarize what we know. We know that the American diet provides us with too many omega-6 EFAs and not enough omega-3 EFAs. We know that it is not enough to simply increase our consumption of omega-3 EFAs, and we know that good health requires a correct omega-6 to omega-3 EFA ratio. We know that the Cloister Workshop has recommended that we consume an omega-6 to omega-3 EFA ratio of 2 to 1. And we know that the villain is trans-fat, not saturated fat.

Reduce Omega-6 EFA Intake

The first step we can take to restore the proper omega-6 to omega-3 ratio in our diet is to reduce our intake of omega-6 rich foods. In Table 17 products are listed according to their omega-6 EFA content in grams per 100 grams edible portion (column 2). Column 3 indicates the omega-3 EFA content and column 4 gives the omega-6 to omega-3 EFA ratio.

Most of the products listed contain omega-6 EFAs in large proportion. Some of them have omega-6 EFAs only. Peanuts and sunflower oil have little or no omega-3 EFAs and thus a very high omega-6 to omega-3 ratio. The low omega-6 EFA content of peanuts and of peanut butter put them in a favorable position at the bottom of the list in Table 16. Peanuts and peanut butter, however, contain several allergens absent in the other omega-6 rich products. We have seen that allergens are substances that trigger an immune response and that the omega-6 EFAs contribute to stimulate an immune response. It should not come as a surprise that peanuts—a combination of allergens and omega-6 EFAs in the same product—have become a prominent food allergen in the U.S.[197]

Three products—soybean oil, wheat germ oil and canola oil—contain enough omega-3 EFAs to give them an acceptable omega-6 to omega-3 ratio. The 2.18 to 1 ratio of canola oil is much better than the 8 to 1 ratio of both soybean oil and wheat germ oil. Canola oil also contains less omega-6 EFAs and more omega-3 EFAs. All of this makes canola oil appear to be the best choice. But beware! Canola oil is a very recently introduced industrial product that lacks a history of safe use by humans over time. It is extracted from rapeseed that has been genetically modified to reduce its natural toxicity. Indeed, rapeseed oil is so toxic that it is used as an insecticide. Did you know that canola oil—the rapeseed oil derivative—is still regulated by the EPA as a pesticide?[198]

At the bottom of the table are four products that deserve our attention: flaxseed oil, lard, olive oil and butter. Of these, flaxseed oil has the highest content of omega-3 EFAs and will be discussed in the next section of this chapter. As for the other three, we can only conclude that these old-fashioned foods are much better candidates than their more recent counterparts for lowering the omega-6 content of our diet. In addition, please note that butter has an omega-6 to omega-3 ratio that exceeds the recommendations of the Cloister Workshop!

Product	Omega-6 EFAs	Omega-3 EFAs	Ratio: Omega-6 to -3
Sunflower Oil	66	0	n-6 only
Corn Oil	58	0.7	83 to 1
Wheat germ Oil	55	6.9	8 to 1
Soybean Oil	51	6.9	8 to 1
Safflower Oil Margarine	45	0	n-6 only
Sesame Oil	41	0.3	138 to 1
Apricot Kernel Oil	29	0	n-6 only
Avocado Oil	29	0	n-6 only
Safflower Seed Oil	28	0.1	253 to 1
Brazil Nuts	26	0.6	384 to 1
Corn Oil Margarine	24	0.4	59 to 1
Sesame Seed Oil	21	0.3	57 to 1
Canola Oil	20	9.3	2.18 to 1
Soybean Oil Margarine	19	1.5	13 to 1
Peanuts	16	0.003	5,333 to 1
Flaxseed Oil	14	60	0.24 to 1
Lard	10	1	10 to 1
Olive Oil	8	0.6	13 to 1
Butter	1.83	1.18	1.5 to 1

Table 17. Foods listed by their omega-6 EFA content in grams per 100 grams edible portion. The second column indicates their omega-3 EFA content, and the third column indicates the ratio of omega-6 to omega-3 EFAs.

Increase Omega-3 EFA Intake

Of all the foods listed in Table 17, flaxseed oil appears to be the only candidate that can really do the job for us of both increasing omega-3 EFAs and decreasing the ratio of omega-6 to omega-3 EFAs. The table shows us that flaxseed oil provides a remarkable 60 grams of omega-3 EFAs per hundred grams and yields an astounding omega-6 to omega-3 EFA ratio of 0.24. So the next question we want to ask is "Will supplementing our diet with flax seed or flaxseed oil be sufficient?"

Until very recently, the answer to this question would have been an unqualified "yes." With flaxseed oil's abundance of omega-3 EFAs we might have assumed that we could easily bring the omega-6 to omega-3 EFA ratio in our diet into balance. But now we know that there is another critical factor that we must take into account: the type of omega-3 EFA involved.

The prevalent scientific opinion used to be that humans could readily make EPA (eicosapentaenoic acid) and DHA (docosahexaenoic acid) from ALA (alpha-linolenic acid). But this has been proven wrong.[199]

> Our capacity to make longer chain omega-3 EFAs by elongation and desaturation of ALA is very limited at best.

In the world of fatty acids, long chains are made from short chains. This is true of the essential fatty acids (EFAs) as well as the non-essential fatty acids. Long chain omega-6 EFAs are made from short chain omega-6 EFAs and long chain omega-3 EFAs are made from short chain omega-3 EFAs. The same elongase and desaturase enzymes participate in turning short chain EFAs into long chain EFAs.

For purposes of illustrating what goes on in the body at the biochemical level, let us imagine a fatty acid synthesis site as having two production lines. Let us call the production line of long chain omega-6 fatty acids "Line 1" and the production line of long chain omega-3 fatty acids "Line 2." Now let us visualize the relationship between the two lines as they compete for the same enzymes in order to each turn their short chain fatty acids into long chain fatty acids. Line 1 and Line 2 are competing for the same elongase and desaturase enzymes. Which line wins . . . which line gets the enzymes? For most Americans it is Line 1, the omega-6 EFA production line.

It was recently discovered that the production line that has the most abundant supply of short chain fatty acids monopolizes the enzymes! This is where our diet tells the tale. People who consume much more of the omega-6 "Line 1" EFA linoleic acid (LA) than they do of the omega-3 "Line 2" EFA alpha-linolenic acid (ALA) have no problem producing the long chain omega-6 EFAs they need to make their omega-6 prostaglandins. However, they have big problems making the long chain omega-3 EFAs they need to produce the prostaglandins that have the opposite and necessary effect of "braking" cell activity—including allaying and reducing the inflammatory response. They have problems because "Line 2" does not have enough short chain omega-3 ALA in order to compete for the enzymes it needs to make its derivative long chain EFAs.

To make matters worse, the long chain omega-3 production line (Line 2) is just a slow production line. Even under the best of nutritional conditions—when the omega-6 to omega-3 ratio is 2 to 1—the conversion of ALA into longer chain omega-3 EFAs occurs only at a very low rate and a very slow pace. It appears that in the best conditions only 15% of the ingested ALA becomes eicosapentaenoic acid (EPA) and only 5% is changed into docosahexaenoic acid (DHA).

The Function of EPA and DHA

These indispensable long chain omega-3 essential fatty acids, EPA and DHA, are the key for many Americans who live in a state of compromised health—wherein every cell of the body is compromised by our diet. How can we reverse this state? By supporting the structure, integrity and function of our cells via EPA and DHA. We must not underestimate the roles they play in helping to regulate our blood lipids and decrease inflammation, maintain the fluidity of our blood and protect our heart rhythm while lowering our blood pressure (Table 18).

Action	EPA	DHA
Increase of HDL cholesterol	yes	yes
Decrease triglycerides	yes	yes
Increase blood clotting	yes	
Stabilize heart rhythm	yes	
Reduce inflammation	yes	yes
Lower blood pressure		yes
CNS growth and maintenance		yes

Table 18. The main effects of EPA and DHA.

The long chain essential fatty acid DHA is also indispensable for brain and nervous system growth and maintenance. For good health we must guarantee that our bodies are well supplied with food and/or supplements containing EPA and DHA!

Increase our Intake of Long Chain Omega-3 EFAs

No pun intended, the long and the short of it is that the only real way to restore our health is to increase our consumption of food and/or supplements that already contain the omega-3 long chain essential fatty acids EPA (eicosapentaenoic acid) and DHA (docosahexaenoic acid). Although it feels like we will never be able to spell—much less say—the names of these essential fatty acids, it is truly worth our while to remember their "nicknames": EPA and DHA. Just repeat them a few times to yourself and they will no longer feel like strangers from a strange land.

What food contains long chain omega-3 EFAs? Fish and cold water fish in particular (Table 19).

Food	ALA	EPA	DHA	Sum of EPA + DHA	Total Omega-3 EFAs	LA	Omega-6 to Omega-3 Ratio
Atlantic Salmon	0.09	0.62	1.29	1.91	2.01	1.05	0.52 to 1
Pacific Herring	0.06	0.97	0.69	1.66	1.72	0.19	0.11 to 1
European Anchovy	0	0.54	0.91	1.45	1.45	0.10	0.07 to 1
Sardine	0.23	0.53	0.86	1.39	1.62	0.12	0.7 to 1
Chinook Salmon	0.09	0.79	0.57	1.36	1.44	0.11	0.07 to 1
Bluefish	0	0.25	0.52	0.77	0.77	0.06	0.08 to 1
Trout	0.11	0.16	0.42	0.58	0.69	0.23	0.3 to 1
Shrimp - mixed	0.01	0.26	0.22	0.48	0.49	0.03	0.06 to 1
Halibut	0.07	0.07	0.29	0.36	0.43	0.03	0.07 to 1
Yellowfin Tuna	0.01	0.04	0.18	0.22	0.23	0.01	0.03 to 1
Atlantic Cod	0.001	0.064	0.12	0.18	0.19	0.005	0.03 to 1

Table 19. Alpha-linolenic acid (ALA), eicosapentaenoic acid (EPA), docosa-hexaenoic acid (DHA), sum of EPA and DHA, total omega-3 fatty acids, linoleic acid (LA) contents per 100 grams and the omega-6 to omega-3 ratio of some foods with high EPA and DHA contents.

Cold ocean fish and fish oils have a great advantage over flax seed and flaxseed oil because the former contain many long chain omega-3 EFAs, which include EPA and DHA, while flaxseed oil contains only the short chain omega-3 EFA alpha-linolenic acid (ALA). Cold ocean fish and fish oils are actually the only reliable natural sources of EPA and DHA. This may change in the near future. Research is already in progress to manipulate plant and terrestrial animals to produce long chain omega-3 EFAs.[200]

Stay Away from Trans Fatty Acids

Trans fatty acids lurk in a multitude of foods and we have seen in chapter 9 that they do not fit in our biochemistry. The bad news is that trans fatty acids are detrimental to health. It was ten years ago that an article in *Lancet*, the leading British medical journal and the equivalent of the *Journal of the American Medical Association (JAMA)*, revealed that the consumption of food rich in trans fatty acids increases the risk of heart and vascular disease, and that the consumption of major sources of trans fatty acids like margarine, cookies and fried food is significantly associated with higher risks of heart and vascular disease.[201] This information has been confirmed by more recent research.[202]

The good news for us is that we can be pro-active consumers. We can limit our consumption of fried foods and know what to look for on food labels. The FDA has ruled that the "Trans Fat" content of foods be listed on all food labels by January 1, 2006.[203] Until then, we can keep our eyes open for three ingredients that are a sure tip-off: "partially hydrogenated vegetable oil," "hydrogenated vegetable oil" and "shortening." To help you solve the mystery of where these trans fatty acids are hiding you can always visit the Web. One site that is particularly informative is the Trans Fatty Acids database from Richard Fang.[204]

Chapter 11

Scarcity of Some Carbohydrates

Many forward-thinking professionals in health and nutrition still talk about carbohydrates as if they were only sources of energy. However, there are carbohydrates that have critical functions other than serving as fuel for the body.

Function of Carbohydrates in Human Biochemistry

Eight carbohydrates have well-defined functions in human biochemistry. What this means is that biochemists have deciphered the roles those eight carbohydrates play in our biochemistry. It does not mean that other carbohydrates have no role in human biochemistry or that their roles are any less important. Over the last few years the roles of an array of carbohydrates in cell and organ structure, cell metabolism, cell communication and immunity have been progressively documented. But the fact remains that there is still much, much more for scientists who specialize in "glycobiology" to discover, and the implications for our health are great.[205,206]

Some of them are simple molecules that—like the glucose molecule[207]—contain only carbon, oxygen and hydrogen atoms. Mannose is an example of one such simple molecule.

Other simple carbohydrate molecules carry an additional group of atoms, such as an *amine* group. An amine group is made of one atom of nitrogen (whose chemical symbol is N) with one or two hydrogen atoms. When a carbohydrate carries an amine group, the suffix "amine" is added to the name of the carbohydrate. For example, glucose with an amine group is called "glucosamine" [208] and galactose with an amine group is called "galactosamine." [209] Another example of a side group found on simple carbohydrates is the *acetyl* group (CH3-COOH), which is a part of the molecule we know of as vinegar. Other simple carbohydrates carry two additional groups. Examples of these would be N-acetyl galactosamine and N-acetyl glucosamine.

Complex Carbohydrates

Carbohydrates become complex carbohydrates in a number of ways. They can form larger molecules made up of successive identical simple carbohydrates. They can be molecules that contain multiple units of different simple carbohydrates. And they can form compounds that combine carbohydrate with other molecules such as lipids (fats), proteins, parts of lipids (fatty acids) or parts of proteins (amino acids). This category of complex carbohydrates is known as "glycoconjugates."

Carbohydrates in Human Biochemistry

In addition to the roles that we have previously discussed, carbohydrates also participate extensively in the structure of our organs and in cell communication.

The Collagen Matrix: Holding Things Together

Complex carbohydrates are essential parts of the structure that gives our organs their strength.[210] Have you ever wondered why the organs in your body don't fall apart? What is it that holds the cells of an organ together, including the nerves and the blood vessels it contains? It is an amazing binding substance—a glycoconjugate—called collagen. Collagen is a matrix that forms a supporting network between the cells, the nerves and the blood vessels. All organs contain collagen, and bone is no exception. However, there is a big difference between the collagen in bone and the collagen in other organs. The difference is that the collagen in bone contains minerals.

Like all molecules in the body, the molecules that comprise the collagen of our organs (including bones) are the objects of a constant turnover. Molecules of collagen are continuously broken down, removed and replaced by new molecules. The constant shift of molecules implies that we have to provide our organs and bones with a continuous supply of building blocks for the maintenance of our collagen. Any shortage of supply will cause a weakening of our organs—their size, strength and ability to do work.

OSTEOPOROSIS REVISITED

Unless we have a sufficient supply of the essential building blocks for the collagen in our bones, our bodies cannot completely restore that collagen matrix. When less collagen is re-built there is less storage space for calcium. Calcium supplementation alone is insufficient to maintain bone integrity. Vertebra may silently collapse under the weight of the body. Other effects can be even more brutal—like a bone fracturing at the slightest strain.

We have all heard or known of people who have taken a tumble and broken their hip. This hip fracture is, regrettably, the most commonplace and spectacular consequence of osteoporosis. It occurs at the top of the thigh bone, known as the femoral neck or epiphysis. A fracture of the femoral neck occurs when that osteoporotic bone experiences the slightest strain that exceeds its strength. When the bone is osteoporotic strain is being placed on it all the time and by nothing more than simply walking around.

Osteoporosis is a very gradual phenomenon—although a fracture occurs in a split second, the conditions that lead up to it take a long time to develop. The strength of the femur's epiphysis diminishes slowly—unnoticed. Unnoticed until ... the moment that the simple strain of walking around exceeds the resistance of the crumbling bone and the femur fractures. First comes the fracture then the fall, in the direction of the broken bone. The fall is the consequence, not the cause, of the fracture.

Cell Communication

Carbohydrates play a pivotal role in our health, particularly our immunity. They accomplish this via the specific tasks they perform in cell communication. We have already looked at how our immune response works—what causes it and what regulates it. We have discussed how the intensity of our immune response closely depends on our diet. Now we will take a closer look at the target recognition aspect of our immune response and see where key carbohydrates from our diet come into play.

THE CELL'S ID

We have already established that all our cells wear identification molecules that protrude from their membranes. By now it will probably not surprise you one bit that these ID molecules are made of glycoconjugates. Specifically, these glycoconjugates that assure the cell's identity are glycoproteins: carbohydrate and protein. The protein part of the glycoprotein is embedded in the cell membrane. The carbohydrate part of the glycoprotein protrudes outwards to the exterior of the cell's membrane (Figure 10).

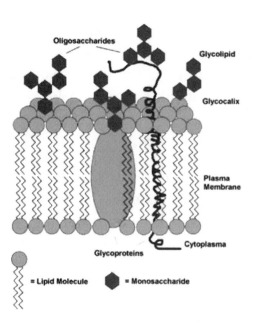

Figure 10. The protein part of glycoprotein is embedded in the cell membrane, with the carbohydrate part of it protruding out to the exterior of the cell's membrane. Courtesy of the GALAB Company.[211]

The carbohydrate part of the glycoprotein makes up the cells' ID tags. By choosing carbohydrates as the tag for our cells, nature made a really sensible decision. Here's why. If nature had chosen to tag cells with amino acids (the constituents of proteins), the number of different possible tags would have been limited. Tagging cells with carbohydrates allows a much greater variety of tags to be created. You see, the number of possible combinations of two or more carbohydrates is much greater than the number of combinations of two or more amino acids. The reason is that a monosaccharide molecule has at least four hydroxyl (-HO) group handles, whereas amino acids have only two handles, and they are selective. One is the amino group (-NH2) and the other is the carboxyl group (-COOH). Two amino acids have only two ways to attach to each other. In contrast, two monosaccharides have 16 different ways that they can attach to each other.

All things being equal, this cell identification system would be foolproof. But that "all things being equal" assumes that nature is provided with all of the ingredients that are required for constructing her vast repertoire of cell tags. Lacking any of these ingredients, errors in construction of cell identification tags occur. It is these errors that then wreak havoc on the immune system. They confuse and disable the immune system's recognition process. If we think of the cell's ID tags as bar codes and the cell's immune system recognition tools as a bar code reader, it is easy to imagine the mess that is caused by any omissions or errors in the bar code tags. Then consider the added confusion that would ensue when the bar code readers themselves (which also contain glycoconjugates) are defective.

IMMUNITY

As we see the "2 + 2" aspects of this equation come together, we are led to an obvious conclusion. If our diet does not provide the variety of carbohydrates that our bodies need to optimally operate all of the biochemical systems that nature has designed for us, we cannot expect to be truly healthy. Carbohydrate deficiency in the diet, leading to errors in the cell bar code and defects in the cell bar code reader, are key factors in the proliferation of immune related conditions. Osteoarthritis offers an example of it.[212]

CHRONIC INFLAMMATION

We have seen that a chronic inflammatory response is part of many conditions. Errors in the structure of molecules comprising carbohydrates contribute to the initiation and to the perpetuation of chronic inflammation as in arthritis[213] and in bladder infection. In bladder infection by *E. coli*, a very common pathogen, the presence of the carbohydrate mannose prohibits the attachment of the germ to the wall of the bladder. This is how mannose supplementation helps people with a chronic bladder infection.[214]

Essential Carbohydrates

Without a doubt we are now alert to the fact that the American diet has an excess of the carbohydrate glucose and fructose. What about others? We know that science has defined the roles of seven others that play critical roles in cell and organ structure as well as cell communication. They are galactose, mannose, xylose, fucose, neuraminic N-acetyl acid, N-acetyl glucosamine and N-acetyl galactosamine.

There are two ways that we can get these 7 essential carbohydrates. One is by having our bodies synthesize them from glucose or fructose. The other is by getting them directly from the food we eat. Let us take a moment to explore the first method.

It is entirely true that our bodies can synthesize these 7 carbohydrates. But the mere fact that our bodies can do so does not mean that internal synthesis is the wisest or most efficient way of acquiring them. Unfortunately, science has operated for too long on the theory that glucose and fructose are the sole carbohydrates we have to get from our food and that our biochemistry will simply synthesize all the others we need.

Fortunately, there is a dawning recognition that this view is simplistic and naïve. Take a look at Table 20 and you will see why. Our bodies must do a lot of work to make these monosaccharide conversions. Every step requires the participation of at least one enzyme, and every enzyme involved must be recruited—or synthesized itself—from somewhere in our biochemistry. A psychologist looking at this process might well call these carbohydrate conversions classical examples of "co-dependence." A tremendous amount of energy is expended to achieve a particular result while there are other, unintended results that also take place. Each one requires a less-than-efficient energy expenditure. Those conversions that entail 7, 8 and 10 steps are indeed long, labor intensive and highly inefficient (Table 20).

Monosaccharides	Enzymatic steps from glucose	Enzymatic steps from fructose
Glucose	3	
Fructose	1	
Galactose	6	7
Mannose	4	3
Xylose	5	6
Fucose	10	9
Neuraminic N-acetyl acid	10	9
N-acetyl glucosamine	7	6
N-acetyl galactosamine	8	7

Table 20. The conversion of a monosaccharide into another may involve up to ten enzymatic steps. (Derived from Food Composition and Nutritional Tables by Souchi, Fachmann Kraut, Stuttgart 1986)

A Far Better Approach.

The good news is that galactose, mannose, xylose, fucose, neuraminic N-acetyl acid, N-acetyl glucosamine and N-acetyl galactosamine are readily absorbable from foods that contain them. They all occur as simple or complex molecules in plant and animal products where they make up the structural components of those foods. The best plant products are fruit and vegetables, other than those that are full of starch.[215] The best animal products are bone, cartilage and organs.[216]

> The fact is that, aside from galactose
> (present in milk and milk products),
> the other carbohydrates with a documented function
> in human biochemistry have become scarce in
> or are missing from the American diet.

The reasons for the absence or scarcity of these carbohydrates in the American diet are the overuse of processed foods and the paucity of fresh fruits and vegetables in the diet of most people.

The Prevalence of Processed Food

Processed foods have created a revolution in human culture. They have revolutionized what we eat, the way we eat and the way we think about food. They have revolutionized food production, and they have revolutionized the marketing of food. They have radically changed population demographics, family lifestyle, individual careers and life choices. And processed foods have changed the culture and content of food itself.

Processed food contains far fewer components than the original food (i.e., the crop as delivered to us by nature) from which it is made. Take flour as an example. Flour is mainly starch, whereas the original grain from which it is made contains several other carbohydrates in addition to minerals, vitamins, other molecules with a nutritive value as well as nonnutritive molecules that our bodies need (such as fiber).

Processed food is presented as "refined" food—and we tend to think better of it because it is refined. We think of it as being more sophisticated, more technologically advanced—better, cleaner, more "American." In reality, refined food is food that has been stripped of many of its health-promoting properties and therefore much of its value. Whole wheat is turned into white flour, whole rice is made into polished rice and potatoes are turned into instant mashed potatoes. A whole host of valuable constituents— including a variety of carbohydrates needed by our biochemistry—are lost in the processing.

The Scarcity of Fresh Fruit and Vegetables

In a country that many consider to be the breadbasket of the world, even the mere notion of a scarcity of fresh fruit and vegetables seems ludicrous. But agricultural production capability is one thing and consumption is another. According to statistics from the U.S. Department of Agriculture, in 2002 Americans consumed just over 100 pounds of fresh fruit and 174 pounds of fresh vegetables per capita (excluding potatoes.) The total of both was just over 274 pounds for that year (Table 21).[217]

	Fresh
Fruit	100.1
Vegetables	174.2
Totals	274.3

Table 21. Per capita consumption of fresh fruit and vegetables in 2002.

When we divide by 365 days a year, it works out that Americans consumed three-quarter (3/4) pound of fresh fruit and vegetables per person per day in 2002.

Reality Check

Our first thought upon seeing these figures might be one of pleasant surprise. Three-quarter pound of fresh fruit and vegetables per day sounds like quite a lot, doesn't it? The unfortunate answer is "Yes, it does." What makes it unfortunate is that Americans fail to realize that fresh fruit and vegetables are what nature intended (and our bodies agree) to be part of the core foundation of a healthy diet, rather than a "healthy" addition to a diet. Thanks to the advent of processed food, our basic concept of food—what constitutes our daily diet—has been turned inside out. We think of fruit and vegetables as colorful and good-for-us side dishes or between meal snacks, rather than the central features of every meal that they ought to be.

So where can we turn for "a reality check"? The best source available to us for a reality check is the World Health Organization (WHO), the international body of the United Nations whose overall stated goal is "to improve public health through healthy eating and physical activity." Their web site tells us the following about WHO's comprehensive "Global Strategy on Diet, Physical Activity and Health" that was endorsed by the World Health Assembly in 2004:

A few largely preventable risk factors account for most of the world's disease burden. Chronic diseases—including cardiovascular conditions, diabetes, stroke, cancers and respiratory diseases—account for 59% of the 57 million deaths annually, and 46% of the global disease burden. This represents a significant change in diet habits and physical activity levels worldwide as a result of industrialization, urbanization, economic development and increasing food market globalization.[218]

Would you agree that this is a singularly strong statement—perhaps even a sweeping indictment—of the status of human health around the world? Would you further agree that the above description fits us Americans to a tee … that it is we Americans who might be "leading the pack" in terms of those preventable risk factors and the chronic diseases that they lead to?

Not surprisingly, our WHO reality check takes us right back to . . . daily servings of fresh fruit and vegetables.

The WHO Recommendation

The World Health Organization recommends a daily intake of 1.1 pounds (500 grams) of fresh fruit and vegetables per person per day. That represents a total consumption per year of 401 pounds. Glancing back at Table 21 we can see that American consumption of fresh fruit and vegetables falls quite short of the WHO recommendation. In fact, our annual consumption is only a little over two-thirds (2/3) of that. Let us refer once again to the WHO web site to better understand why they recommend what they do:

Low fruit and vegetable intake is among the top 10 risk factors contributing to attributable mortality, according to evidence presented in World Health Report 2003. Fruits and vegetables as part of the daily diet could help prevent major noncommunicable diseases (NCD) such as cardiovascular diseases and certain cancers. Eating a variety of vegetables and fruits clearly ensures an adequate intake of most micronutrients, dietary fibres and a host of essential non-nutrient substances.[219]

Our bodies need the micronutrients, dietary fibers and essential non-nutrient substances that are contained in fresh fruit and vegetables.

Why on earth are we starving our bodies and compromising our health by replacing fresh fruits and vegetables with processed foods that simply do not contain everything we need to be healthy? This strategy that underlies the American diet does not make any sense!

What We Can Do

Increase Our Intake of Fresh Fruit and Vegetables

Once again we can turn to the World Heath Organization to decipher what we should do. WHO breaks down their daily recommendation into recommended servings per day for different age groups. They recommend that children under the age of 6 have 2 servings of fruit and 3 servings of vegetables per day. The recommendation for children over the age of 6, for teenage girls and for women is 3 servings of fruit and 4 servings of vegetables per day. Teenage boys and men should have 4 servings of fruit and 5 servings of vegetables per day (Table 22).[220]

	Fruits	Vegetables	Totals
Children, age 2 to 6	2	3	5
Children over age 6, Teenage girls, Most women	3	4	7
Teenage boys and most men	4	5	9

Table 22. WHO recommendation for fruit and vegetable consumption according to age and gender.

Looked at from a larger perspective according to their goals and guidelines, the WHO considers increasing our consumption of fruits and vegetables to be the most cost effective approach to reducing the frequency of non-communicable diseases (NCD) while lowering the cost of healthcare.[221]

It is generally agreed upon that NCD are linked primarily to bad eating habits, alcohol and smoking, and reduced physical activity. According to the World Health Organization, all type 2 diabetes, 80% of coronary heart disease and 33% of cancers could be prevented by changes in lifestyle factors such as diet, weight maintenance and physical activity.[222]

In a presentation in 2000, Dr. Puska, director of the Non-Communicable Disease Prevention and Health Promotion Department of the World Health Organization in Geneva, emphasized that their main strategy for preventing NCD is to encourage people to increase their fruit and vegetable consumption to recommended levels.[223, 224]

Dr. Puska cites the following factors as the main obstructions to the dietary prevention of the non-communicable diseases:

1. The myth that NCD are the consequence of aging

2. Low public visibility for the results of prevention

3. Little understanding of the prevention potential

4. Powerful commercial interest blocking new policies

5. Routine health professional preference for curative care

6. Inertia in making changes

Where Does This Leave Us?

Our foods are increasingly processed and the percentage of our diet that is made up of whole, nutrient-rich food continues to decline. The indications are clear: we must increase our intake of fresh fruit and vegetables.

Chapter 12

An Excess of Additives and Pesticides

The next time you are in the produce department at the grocery store take a close look at a banana box. The label will read something like this: "Imazalil and/or thiabendazole or azoxystrobin applied to maintain freshness." On a chocolate bar wrapper you will see "maltitol, inulin, soya lecithin and flavors" listed among other ingredients on the label. An entire laundry list of additives is what you will see printed in small type on the nicely designed turkey dinner package you can find in your supermarket freezer. This frozen dinner of turkey breast with stuffing, mashed potatoes and gravy, green beans and cranberries lists the following additives: "Ammonium sulfate, artificial flavors, autolyzed yeast extract, BHT, calcium caseinate, sodium caseinate, calcium propionate, calcium sulfate, caramel color, carrageenan, chicken flavor, dextrose, dicalcium phosphate, disodium dihydrogen pyrophosphate, disodium guanylate, disodium inosinate, emulsified soy lecithin, enzyme modified butter fat, flavor, fructose, gelatin, citric acid, high fructose corn syrup, hydrolyzed corn protein, maltodextrin, modified food starch, monocalcium phosphate, monosodium glutamate, partially hydrogenated soybean oil, polyglycerol esters of fatty acids (emulsifiers), sodium acid pyrophosphate, sodium bisulfite, soy lecithin, soy protein isolate, TBH, whey and yeast extract."

The chemicals listed on the banana box are pesticides. The chemicals in the chocolate bar and in the frozen turkey dinner are food additives. Because of the fact that they are regulated and because pesticides and food additives are used so extensively in our food supply, much of the time we may even forget that they are there. So before discussing their effect on our health let us go back to Square One, as we call it, and take a look at the definitions of both of these categories of substances and their regulation.

Definition

What Is a Pesticide?

The U.S. Environmental Protection Agency (EPA) defines a pesticide as any substance or mixture of substances intended for preventing, destroying, repelling, or mitigating any pest.[225] The EPA warns that by their very nature, most pesticides create some risk of harm to humans, animals, or the environment because they are designed to kill or otherwise adversely affect living organisms.

What Is an Additive?

The U.S. Federal Food, Drug & Cosmetic Act (FDCA) defines an additive as a substance that is added to food to improve it and is safe.[226]

U.S. Regulations

Pesticides and food additives are regulated.

Pesticides

In the U.S. the Environmental Protection Agency (EPA) and the individual states (usually the Department of Agriculture within each state) register or license pesticides for use. The EPA receives its authority to register pesticides under the Federal Insecticide, Fungicide and Rodenticide Act (FIFRA). The states are authorized to regulate pesticides under FIFRA and under their state pesticide laws. States may place more restrictive requirements on pesticides than the EPA. Pesticides must be registered both by the EPA and the state before distribution.[227]

Food Additives

The Federal Food, Drug, and Cosmetics Act of 1938 gave the Food and Drug Administration (FDA) authority over food and food ingredients. The Food Additives Amendment of 1958 requires that the FDA approve a food additive for use. However, two groups of substances are exempted from the food additive regulation process:

1. All substances that the FDA had determined were safe for use in specific food prior to the 1958 amendment were designated as prior-sanctioned substances. Examples in this group are sodium nitrite and potassium nitrite, which are used to preserve luncheon meat.

2. The "generally recognized as safe" or "GRAS" substances. GRAS substances are those whose use is generally recognized by experts as safe, based on their long history or extensive use in food or based on published scientific evidence. Examples of GRAS substances are salt,

pepper, vinegar, baking powder and monosodium glutamate (MSG). Salt, pepper, vinegar, baking powder are GRAS substances because they were routinely added to food for many, many years before the agency was created. This is true for salt, pepper and vinegar. Monosodium glutamate, however, is another story. We will see in a moment that its inclusion in the GRAS list is enough to make us question the validity of the whole listing process.

Pesticides Used on Food

In this discussion we are not addressing the use of pesticides on food crops. What we are talking about is the direct application of pesticides to the foods themselves after they are harvested. Fruits and vegetables in particular are treated with pesticides as they move from grower to market. The primary reason for this pesticide use on fruits and vegetables is to extend their shelf life.

There are three primary pesticides used for this purpose: imazalil, thiabendazole and azoxystrobin. All of them are designed to stop any fungal growth that might alter the quality of the food. Pesticides are applied to all kinds of fruits and vegetables by spraying, waxing or dipping. Imazalil is used on bananas, pears and tomatoes, among other produce. Thiabendazole is widely used on fruits. Azoxystrobin is one of a class of 32 pesticides. It is used extensively on apples, tomatoes, lettuce, strawberries and grapes.

One method by which pesticide is applied to melons is to drench them in a solution of the product. Another method is to wax the melons with a mixture of the same.

According to an investigation by the Pesticide Management Unit of the Food and Agriculture Organization of the United Nations the flesh of melons treated by both drenching and waxing with a pesticide contains residues of it.

Is this pesticide residue harmless to the humans who eat the treated melons? The Institute of Food Safety and Toxicology of Denmark's Veterinary and Food Administration has conducted research on 22 pesticides. They have found that 7 of these 22 pesticides affect humans by inhibiting the production of some of the hormones produced by the adrenal glands.[228] In an animal experiment, pesticides were also found to be toxic for liver cells.[229]

Many people believe that peeling a fruit or vegetable removes all of the pesticide residue clinging to it. Beware! Pesticides can and do penetrate through the skin and into the flesh.

In view of the general recommendation to wash and rinse fruits and vegetables in order to remove the pesticide residues, it is assumed that most of the residues present are removed during that process and that any remaining residue is safe for human consumption. But this assumption overlooks an important fact. **The residue levels that are considered safe apply to each specific chemical separately.**

But let us think about this. Chances are that we rarely encounter chemical pesticides one at a time. In the course of a single meal or snack we may be exposed to one or more of them, in the course of a day to several (many?) more. And over the course of a week, who knows how many? So our exposure would be cumulative, not discrete.

There is another question to be considered. Although the subject of pesticide residue in whole fruits and vegetables has at least been broached, what do we know about the residue in fruit and vegetable juices?... After all, pesticides are soluble in water.

Another consideration with potentially enormous implications is the effect of pesticides on children. Because children are smaller than adults and their organs are still developing, there is good reason to question whether they are more vulnerable to the effects of fungicides and other pesticides. Do the same "safe levels" apply to them?

Additives in Food

All processed foods contain additives.[230] Some food additives may be beneficial, others have no deleterious effect, still others are detrimental to health.[231]

Why Are Food Additives Used?

Additives are put into foods to extend their shelf life, to make them look more appealing, to modify their consistency and to enhance their taste. That is quite a gamut of alterations when you think about it! Given the endless possibilities of ways that food can be altered, it should be no surprise that the FDA lists more than 2,000 substances that are added to food in the U.S.[232]

Let us familiarize ourselves with some of the more commonly used additives and explore what is known about them, including claims from their manufacturers and research findings that may be in disagreement with those claims.

Aspartame

Aspartame is an artificial product that breaks down in the intestine into aspartic acid, phenylalanine, and methanol. Aspartic acid and phenylalanine are naturally occurring amino acids, and methanol is a toxic substance. Aspartame is between 160 and 200 times sweeter than sugar. Aspartame is added to breath mints, cocoa mixes, soft drinks, candy, cereals, coffee beverages, instant breakfasts, gelatin desserts, sugar-free chewing gum, frozen desserts and dinners, many beverages, toppings and yogurt. Aspartame also exists as a stand-alone sweetener in those innocent-looking little packs on every restaurant/café table.

The producers of aspartame say their product is safe.[233] There is much controversy about the research done by the producers,[234] and several researchers have a different opinion, claiming aspartame causes seizures,[235] severe migraines,[236] eye damage and vision loss, confusion, tremors, depression, anxiety attacks and insomnia. [237]

In January 2005, a Scirus search with the key words "aspartame toxicity" yielded 2,867 publications.[238] The toxicity of aspartame is attributed to the chemicals resulting from its breakdown. The chemical of most interest is formaldehyde. In animal experiments, formaldehyde has caused cell damage at a concentration equivalent to what would be seen in humans after intensive use of the product.[239] Given the consumption patterns of Americans when it comes to the kinds of foods that contain aspartame (e.g., soft drinks, coffee beverages, candy, chewing gum, sweeteners), chances are that people are repeatedly ingesting this food additive. Clearly, one should stay away from products containing aspartame.

Autolyzed Yeast Extract

Autolyzed yeast extracts are manufactured from the baker's yeast, *Saccharomyces cerevisiae*. Yeast extracts are used as a source of proteins. Autolyzed yeast extracts can contain up to 77% proteins. However, the autolyzing process of the yeast proteins yields monosodium glutamate, which is, like aspartame, an additive to avoid. (See discussion further on in this chapter.)

Bromate

Potassium bromate is a chemical that improves the baking characteristics of flours.

Bromate was first found to cause tumors in rats in 1982. Subsequent studies on rats and mice confirmed that it causes tumors of the kidney, thyroid and other organs. Instead of banning bromate, the FDA—with only partial success—has urged bakers to voluntarily stop using it.

Potassium bromate was banned in several European countries after studies found that it induces kidney tumors in rats. The Center for Science in the Public Interest (CSPI) has petitioned the Food and Drug Administration (FDA) to prohibit the use of potassium bromate in baking. CSPI charged that the FDA has known for years that bromate causes cancers in laboratory animals but has failed to ban it.[240] California, however, has already banned the use of the additive declaring bromate a carcinogen under the state's Proposition 65. California bakers have switched to bromate-free flour.[241]

BHT

BHT is short for butylated hydroxytoluene. BHT is an antioxidant. As other antioxidants, it protects against free radicals by reducing the oxidation rate of food components that otherwise might change the color and/or the taste of the food product. There is some concern after the discovery that the metabolites of BHT cause lung tumors in laboratory animals.[242] We do not yet know to what extent this finding applies to humans. However, it is a reason to avoid products that contain BHT.

Calcium Caseinate

According to its producers calcium caseinate is a high quality milk protein product manufactured from pasteurized skimmed milk through acid precipitation of the casein followed by neutralization and drying. However, there may be a hidden ingredient in calcium caseinate that can be problematic for many people. Calcium caseinate may contain monosodium glutamate. (See discussion further on in this chapter.)

Calcium Propionate

Calcium propionate is used in bakery products as a mold inhibitor. Calcium propionate has been linked with behavioral changes of inattention, irritability, restlessness and sleep disturbance in children.[243] Of concern are both the amount of bread that children consume as well as the concentration of the preservative used in bread. Calcium propionate has also been linked to an increased incidence of migraine in adults.[244]

Calcium Sulfate

Calcium sulfate is used in human food as well as in animal feed. It is also known in the manufacturing world as gypsum or plaster. Approximately 197,000 tons of gypsum are used annually in the United States as a food binder. Because it readily absorbs moisture and hardens quickly, calcium sulfate has been known to cause intestinal obstruction in humans.

Some producers of calcium sulfate claim that it is a good source of calcium for humans. However, the calcium contributed by calcium sulfate is unlikely to substantially increase our total intake of calcium.

Caramel Color

Color has always played a vitally important role in food selection and acceptance. The color of a food can be the deciding factor in its popularity. Many people are quite surprised—if not incredulous—when they learn that a favorite food is not "naturally" the color that they think it is. Cheddar cheese, for example, is naturally white, just like the milk from which it is made. The yellow or orange color we associate with cheddar cheese is created by the addition of a food colorant.

Caramel color gives food a color that can range from light yellow to reddish and dark browns. The sugars initially undergo dehydration and then condensation or polymerization into complex molecules of varying molecular weight. Lightly colored, pleasant-tasting caramel flavors are produced in the initial stages, but as the reaction continues more high-molecular-weight color bodies are produced, the flavor characteristics become more bitter, and the sulfite content increases.

Caramel color is widely used in beverages and baked goods. In fact, caramel color accounts for more than 90 percent by weight of all the colors added to foods.

When it is produced under high heat and pressure, caramel color may contain **sulfites**. Sulfites may not be a problem for many people, but for millions of Americans sulfites pose a real health concern by exacerbating inflammatory response. After dozens of people died from anaphylactic shock after eating at salad bars, the FDA banned sulfites from that use in 1986. Today, salad bars are safe, but the use of sulfites as preservatives grows as American food habits evolve.

Caramel color prepared by ammonia process has been associated with blood toxicity in rats and with ADHD in children.[245]

Carrageenans

Carrageenans are natural molecules made of chains of galactose. Carrageenan is a collective term for polysaccharides extracted from red seaweeds.

More than six hundred years ago, Irish moss was first used in Carraghen on the south Irish coast for medicinal and food purposes. There, Irish moss was especially known for its unique property of jelling milk. It was also used in a similar way on the coasts of Normandy and Brittany in France. With bleached lichen or "goémon blanc" (blanc-mange), flans were made simply by cooking seaweed in milk.[246]

Carrageenans are used as jelling and thickening agents in the food industry, as a binder in cooked meats and sausages, and as a thickener in pudding. Depending upon how they are processed, carrageenans may or may not contain monosodium glutamate.

Flavoring Agents

Flavoring agents cover the gamut from naturally-occurring substances to laboratory-made chemicals. Hundreds of flavoring agents that come directly from nature (such as aloe, artichoke and sassafras) are probably safe based on historical use. (Please note the word "probably.") Many hundreds more that are found in food products on our supermarket shelves are made from artificial molecules. The challenge posed to the consumer who wants to be well informed is that the companies that produce these foods do not have to disclose the composition of their flavoring formulas.

Both natural and artificial flavoring agents may contain monosodium glutamate or hydrolyzed vegetable protein.

Fructose and High Fructose Corn Syrup

Fructose is a monosaccharide that is approximately 75% sweeter than sugar. For this reason, fructose and fructose products are frequently substituted for sucrose. High fructose corn syrup (HFCS) is made from hydrolyzed corn starch. Starch contains sequences of glucose molecules attached to each other. Hydrolysis breaks the chemical bonds between the glucose molecules, then the enzyme invertase is introduced to change the glucose into fructose, creating high fructose corn syrup. Although HFCS is made from corn starch (glucose) it contains fructose only. HFCS retains moisture better, blends well with flavoring agents, is sweeter than and has a lower viscosity than sugar.

High fructose corn syrup consumption has dramatically increased since it was first introduced. It has largely replaced the ordinary sugar that was previously used in soft drinks and many other foods because it is cheaper. More than one third of all the refined sugar Americans consume is high fructose corn syrup.

> Fructose and HFCS are worse offenders than glucose in producing AGEs (advanced glycation end products—a primary factor in chronic inflammation) and in elevating cholesterol and triglyceride levels.

Hydrolyzed Proteins (Vegetable Protein, Plant Proteins)

Hydrolyzed Protein (HP) is made from a variety of foods (such as soybeans, corn, wheat, or milk whey) that are chemically broken down by acid hydrolysis. It is used extensively as a flavor enhancer in processed foods. Hydrolyzed vegetable protein (HVP) has come to be used as a significant source of protein in manufactured foods—both vegetarian and non-vegetarian food products alike.

> Hydrolyzed protein product may contain monosodium glutamate.

Inulin

Inulin is an example of a potentially beneficial food additive. Inulin has a mildly sweet taste and has filling properties like starch. Inulin is added to food to promote color retention and to preserve freshness. Inulin could be considered a health booster because it is not absorbed yet it promotes the proliferation of useful bacteria in the colon.

Reaction to inulin, even the naturally occurring inulin in such foods as asparagus, garlic, onion and leek, has been noted in some people.[247]

Lecithin

Lecithin is another example of a potentially beneficial additive. Lecithin is a fat-like molecule that is produced by our livers every day. Lecitihin is needed by every cell in the body and is a key building block of cell membranes. As an additive in food, lecithin is a surface-active additive with emulsifying and dispersing properties.

Maltitol

Maltitol is used in food as a sweetener, humectant, stabilizer and bulking agent. Maltitol is hydrogenated high maltose-glucose syrup, about 90 percent as sweet as sucrose (table sugar). Because maltitol does not absorb water from the air, it is stable under heating and has a high melting point.[248] However, because maltitol is poorly absorbed in the human GI tract and is readily broken down by gut bacteria, it may cause diarrhea and flatulence.

Modified Starch

Modified starch, also known as modified food starch, is used as a thickening agent. Starch does not dissolve in cold water and chemists have modified starch to increase its solubility. It may cause diarrhea.

Monosodium Glutamate

The amino acid monosodium glutamate (MSG) brings out the flavor in many foods. While that may sound like a treat for our taste buds, there are drawbacks to consuming MSG. First, its flavor-enhancing properties allow food processors to reduce the amount of real food ingredients in their foods—for example, the amount of chicken product in chicken soup. Second, for over 30 years people have reported that consuming MSG has caused them to experience a variety of unpleasant physical symptoms. Because MSG was once a staple in Chinese restaurant cooking, the effect was dubbed the "Chinese Restaurant Syndrome."

Several food additives always contain glutamate: Autolyzed yeast extract, calcium caseinate, hydrolyzed flour, hydrolyzed vegetable protein, plant protein extract, and sodium caseinate. Many other food additives may contain MSG, such as bouillon, broth, carrageenan, malt extract and flavoring, soy and whey protein concentrate.

There are some loopholes in the FDA regulations. The regulations do not require manufacturers to mention the constituents of the ingredients on their labels. "Broth" can be mentioned without adding that it contains autolyzed yeast extract, sodium caseinate or other potential sources of glutamate.

There is a large body of evidence that glutamate and aspartame are toxic molecules. Whether their exposure comes from Chinese restaurant food or from one or more food additives in a nearly infinite variety of prepared or packaged foods, many people react to MSG and their sensitivity can range from extremely mild to severe. The physical symptoms attributed to MSG consumption include headache, dry mouth, nausea, weakness, burning sensation in the back of neck and forearms, wheezing, changes in heart rate and difficulty breathing. Some people claim to be sensitive to very small amounts of MSG, but no good studies have been done to determine just how little MSG can cause a reaction in the most sensitive people. In his book *Excitotoxins: The Taste that Kills* Dr. Russell L. Blaylock, a practicing neurosurgeon, describes how monosodium glutamate as well as other products like aspartame can disturb brain and nerve function in many people.[249,250]

In the 1960s it was discovered that large amounts of MSG fed to infant mice destroyed nerve cells in the brain. After that research was publicized, public pressure forced companies that manufacture baby food to stop adding MSG to their products.

Despite this change, glutamate is still listed as a "generally recognized as safe" or GRAS substance.

Glutamate is included in the GRAS ("generally recognized as safe") list. Recall the FDA's definition of what qualifies substances to be included on this list: "generally recognized as safe, based on their long history or extensive use in food or based on published scientific evidence."

We believe glutamate does not belong to the GRAS list and here is why: Glutamate is the active ingredient of the sea vegetable kombu used in Japan for centuries as a food spice and food flavor enhancer. Kombu has a long history of safe use and could be added to the GRAS list. As a stand-alone synthetic additive, however, glutamate has no long history or extensive use in food. It was only recently discovered. Furthermore, the published scientific evidence of its safety is challenged by numerous publications saying the opposite.

Like kombu, pepper has a long history of safe use as a food spice and food flavor enhancer. Pepper is rightfully on the GRAS list. However, piperine—the active component of pepper—is not on the GRAS list and for a good reason. Piperine, like glutamate, has no safety record derived from a long history or extensive use in food or based on published scientific evidence.[251]

To sum up, kombu and pepper are examples of additives that should be on the GRAS list. Glutamate and piperine are additives that do not qualify for and should not be on the GRAS list.

Partially Hydrogenated Vegetable Oil

Vegetable oils are hydrogenated to extend their shelf life, unless they are labeled "cold pressed" or "unrefined." Hydrogenated oils—even "partially hydrogenated" oils— always contain trans fatty acids. Furthermore, most vegetable oils also contain omega-6 EFAs and omega-3 EFAs in very unfavorable ratios, as you will recall from chapter 10. Although their argument is obsolete, the vegetable oil industry still presents vegetable oils as a healthy alternative to saturated fat.

Phosphoric Acid

Phosphoric acid is used as an acidifier in soft drinks. This is a great idea for the soft drink manufacturers because it stabilizes and increases the shelf life of their product. However, our bodies might not agree. Soft drinks can upset the fragile acid-alkaline balance of the stomach and small intestines. In addition, the added phosphorus from the phosphoric acid can skew the optimal calcium-to-phosphorus ratio required for healthy bones.

At the 2003 annual meeting of the American Society for Bone and Mineral Research, Katherine Tucker, Ph.D., of Tufts University said that daily consumption of soft drinks containing phosphoric acid may lower bone density.[252] Research over the last 10 years points toward a strong and increasing association between cola beverage consumption and bone fractures in girls. Boys are also at higher risk for bone fractures when their overall calorie intake is low.[253]

Saccharin

Saccharin is about 300 times sweeter than sugar. For over a century saccharin has been used to sweeten foods and beverages without calories or carbohydrates. In 1903 the fledgling company Coca-Cola began receiving shipments of saccharin from another new company, Monsanto, which had been founded for the purpose of producing saccharin. The use of saccharin was considerable during the sugar shortages of the two world wars, particularly in Europe. Today, saccharin has been almost entirely replaced by aspartame in soft drinks as well as many other foods. In 1977, because animal studies had linked saccharin with bladder cancer, the product was banned until December 2000.[254] Today some people suggest that saccharin was subjected to much more rigorous scrutiny than its replacement, aspartame.[255]

Sucralose

Sucralose is 600 times sweeter than sugar but has little or no calorie value. Sucralose is used in baked foods, in drinks, and as a tabletop sweetener. Sucralose is made from sucrose (the table sugar) by substituting three hydroxyl groups (OH) of the molecule for chlorine atoms (Cl).[256]There is controversy about the safety of sucralose. Some researchers claim it is perfectly safe.[257] Others have their doubts.[258]

Multiple Chemical Sensitivity

Multiple Chemical Sensitivity (MCS) is a syndrome in which multiple symptoms reportedly occur with low levels of chemical exposure. Although scientific studies have yet to confirm the cause of MCS, it is widely thought to be caused by a phenomenon known as "synergy" or "synergism." Synergism is the simultaneous, combined activity of separate elements in such a way that, together, they have greater total effect than the sum of their individual effects. Synergy is the subject of abundant warnings in the *Physicians' Desk Reference*, giving contraindications for the use of one drug with another because the side effects from mixing them are recognized to be greater than the side effects from the individual drugs put together. However, it was not until the introduction of the "Gulf War Syndrome" that the concept of synergism was applied to multiple simultaneous chemical exposures.[259]

This author hypothesizes that the same kind of chemical synergism may be taking its toll on the health of Americans via exposure to the multiple additives and pesticide residues in our foods.

What We Can Do

We can take a number of pro-active steps to avoid consuming the pesticides and food additives that are found in so many of our foods.

1. Buy organically grown fresh fruits and vegetables whenever possible.

2. Wash and peel other fresh fruits and vegetables.

3. Read the labels on all processed food that we are

thinking of buying and stay away from foods containing any of the dangerous additives we have discussed or any foods that bear a "laundry list" of additives on their label.

Additionally, we can consider augmenting our diet with the following supplements that have been shown to protect against the effects of pesticides and additives on brain and brain function: acetyl-L-carnitine, carotenoids, coenzyme Q10, flavonoids, magnesium, N-acetyl-l-cysteine (NAC), phosphotidylserine, vitamin C, vitamin E, the vitamins of the B group and zinc.

Chapter 13

An Excess of Calories

A calorie is a unit of energy. The value of one calorie is the amount of energy it takes to raise the temperature of one gram of water by one degree on the Celsius scale. What has this raising of temperature to do with food? The number of calories in a given amount of food tells us the amount of energy that our bodies can extract from that food. Technically speaking, this unit of energy is called a "kilocalorie" and is often notated as *kcal*. But in popular usage we have shortened it to "calorie."

Calories in Food

Food stores calories in various amounts. When our bodies burn them for fuel, carbohydrates and proteins yield about 4 calories per gram. Fats yield 9 calories per gram. These numbers are the calorie contents of pure proteins, pure carbohydrates and pure fat.

Most of our food, however, contains proteins, carbohydrates and fats mixed together in variable proportions, along with water and other molecules that may or may not have important functions in human biochemistry. But like water these other components have no caloric value.

As we are already aware—and no one as much as a dieter—foods differ greatly in their calorie content. Table 23 gives a comparison of the calorie content of 100 gram portions of several different foods. As you look at the table, notice where the calories come from in each of them.

As you can see, oils and fats contain no carbohydrates and no proteins. In oils and fats, all the calories come from fat. Sugar contains no fat and no protein and its 387 calories come from carbohydrate alone. In other foods, the calories come in various proportions from protein, carbohydrate and fat (Table 23).

Food (100 grams)	Total calorie	Percent from Fat	Percent from Protein	**Percent from Carbohydrate**
Oils and Fats	850-990	100	0	0
Sugar	387	0	0	100
Walnuts	654	83	8	9
Cheddar Cheese	403	72	26	1
Brown Long Rice	370	7	7	86
Whole Wheat Bread	246	14	15	71
Chinook Salmon	187	52	48	0
Egg	158	61	37	3
Apple	59	5	1	93

Table 23. The numbers in the table come from the World's Online Culinary Encyclopedia and Nutritional Database. The database contains a massive amount of nutritional information on tens of thousands of food items.[260]

Calories in Human Biochemistry

We use the energy we extract from our food for our basic needs and for our daily activities.

Your Basic Needs

You use energy no matter what you are doing—even when you are sleeping. The amount of calories you need for your basic needs is called your Basal Metabolic Rate (BMR). It is the minimum number of calories you require to stay alive and to keep your basic metabolism functioning. BMR varies with gender, age, height and body weight. For example, a 30-year-old woman who is 5 feet 6 inches tall and weighs 130 pounds needs about 1,394 calories per day. A man of the same age, weight and height would need slightly more, about 1,521 calories per day. Since the BMR varies with gender, age, height and body weight you have to look at several tables to calculate it. A far easier and more efficient way to determine your BMR is to get on the Web and let your computer do it for you.[261]

Your Daily Activity

While BMR is the calories your body needs while at rest, you also need calories to fuel your body during your daily activities. The total amount of calories you need per day is the sum of the calories used to maintain your BMR plus an amount that varies according to your level of physical activity. As a general rule, someone involved in a high performance physical training program needs about 1,000 calories more than a sedentary person (Table 24).[262]

		Female - 30 yr. old 5 ft. 6 in. 130 lbs.	Male - 30 yr. old 5 ft. 6 in. 130 lbs.
Basal Metabolic Rate		**1,394**	**1,521**
Activity level	Very Light	1,763	1,793
	Light	1,897	1,942
	Moderate	2,032	2,092
	Heavy	2,166	2,241
	Very Heavy	2,301	2,390
	Sport	2,435	2,540
	Heavy Training	2,570	2,689

Table 24. Example of daily calorie need for BMR and for various levels of activity.

How It Works

We need to get from our food the amount of calories equal to what our bodies require for our basic needs plus what we expend for our daily activities.[263] It is a simple equation.

But we can run into problems if our calorie intake does not meet our expenditure demand or if there is an imbalance in the opposite direction.

Coping with Calorie Shortage

What happens when our food intake does not supply the amount of calories we need? Borrowing from the language of computers, you can say that our metabolism simply shifts into an underlying "default setting" that it knows well. Thanks to the intelligence of evolution our bodies are well equipped to confront a scarcity of calories. You see, early humans and their ancestors had to struggle to find food and often faced starvation conditions. For them, a well-developed ability to survive shortages of food was an evolutionary necessity. Among the many other attributes that have been handed down to us, we have inherited that capacity from our ancestors. Our bodies are designed to find the calories we need to meet our basic needs. If those calories are not available as food from an outside source then they are found internally. Our bodies meet their basic metabolic needs by using our own fat and muscles for fuel. In addition, during severe calorie shortage the body's basic metabolism is reduced to the essential minimum and drops below the former basic needs level.

Coping with Calorie Excess

Because early humans and their ancestors frequently had to struggle to find food a secondary favorable evolutionary adaptation occurred. The body developed a strong ability to rapidly store a temporary excess of food in the form of body fat. The actual genetic make-up of humanity is the result of exposure to extreme food supply fluctuation over hundreds of thousands of years—exposure to both the hardship of calorie shortages and the bounty of short periods of calorie abundance.

> Because we are designed to cope with the fluctuations between times of temporary calorie shortage and short periods of abundance, we are ill equipped to handle the ceaseless abundance of calories in the American diet.

Excess Calories in the American Diet

It may surprise you to discover that the current abundance of calories in the American diet is only a recent phenomenon. It is an indisputable fact that the size of food portions has increased dramatically in the U.S. over the last 30 years. Portion sizes began to grow in the 1970s, rose more in the 1980s, and continue to grow. But this increase is not a worldwide phenomenon, and if you have traveled outside of the U.S. you can certainly attest to this yourself. In other countries food portions in restaurants, "serving sizes" in cookbooks, and individually packaged meals in grocery stores are smaller than in the U.S.[264]

Here in the U.S. the size of food servings has been beset by its own kind of runaway inflation that makes our economy look tame. Foods that once came in one size only are now offered in a family of size offerings, and the one-size-only size has become the "small" portion. Other family members are designated by names like "large" and "supersize," "grande" and "vente" or "double" and "triple." A hamburger that weighed 5.7 ounces twenty years ago now weighs in at 7 ounces and contains 100 more calories. Soft drinks that were once 13 ounces are now up to 20 ounces, with an increase of about 50 calories.

When it was first imported into the U.S. the original Polish bagel weighed 1.5 ounces. The American bagel now weighs in at 4 to 4.5 ounces. A French croissant in France is about 15 inches in circumference, but in the U.S. it is 28 inches. A quesadilla in the U.S. is now about 10 inches long. In Mexico it is still only 5 inches. Guess what comes along with every increase in size? . . . A corresponding increase in calories, of course—96 for the croissant, 234 for the bagel, and 660 for the quesadilla (Table 25).[265]

Food	Original size	Calories	Actual size	Calories
Bagel	1.5 ounce	116	4 to 4.5 ounces	350
Croissant	1 ounce	174	1.5 to 2 ounces	270
Quesadilla	5 inches	540	10 inches	1,200

Table 25. Evolution of size and calorie content of some foods. Data published by the American Institute for Cancer Research.

How Excess Calories Affect Our Health

There is a growing consensus among researchers that larger food portions and their excess calories contribute to the increasing prevalence of overweight and obesity in the U.S. population.

In 1994 R. J. Kuczmarski from the Division of Health Examination Statistics at the U.S. Centers for Disease Control and Prevention published an article in the *Journal of the American Medical Association* (*JAMA*) describing the substantial increase in overweight among U.S. adults.[266] In 2002 an article by K. M. Flegal from the same agency suggested that the prevalence of obesity and overweight was continuing to rise.[267] In 2004, C. L. Johnson confirmed the trend and identified unhealthy diets and sedentary behaviors as the primary causes of deaths attributable to obesity.[268]

Overweight and Obesity Revisited

Overweight and obesity are increasing in the U.S. and the most recent reports suggest the trend is accelerating.[269] Overweight is defined by a Body Mass Index (BMI) equal to or greater than 25. Obesity is defined by a Body Mass Index equal to or greater than 30. Table 26 presents a more detailed scale.

Weight Classification	**Body Mass Index**
Underweight	Less than 18.5
Normal	18.5 - 24.9
Overweight	25 - 29.9
Obesity I	30 - 34.9
Obesity II	35 - 39.9
Extremely obese (III)	40 and over

Table 26. The weight classifications and their body mass indexes.

What Is Body Mass Index?

Body Mass Index (BMI) is one way of determining our nutritional status. It is a measurement that uses height and weight to determine the fat content of our bodies. BMI can be used to indicate how much risk a person has of developing certain health problems.

Calculating the BMI

Body mass index can be calculated by dividing your weight in pounds by the square of the height in inches and multiplying the result by 7.03. For example, a person who weighs 175 pounds and is 5 feet 11 inches (71 inches) tall has a BMI of 24.4.

One can also calculate the BMI using centimeters and kilograms by dividing the weight in kilograms by the square of the height in meters. For example, a person who weighs 80 kilograms and is 1.80 meters tall has a BMI of 24.5.[270, 271]

Of course, body mass index is not the only indicator of health, but it is a useful tool for determining whether your body weight may be affecting your health and putting you at risk. The older approaches to BMI that use 30 years of age as a reference standard as well as obsolete formulas have been superceded by newer and better ones. For example, the web site of Steven B. Halls, M.D.[272] contains a much more detailed concept of BMI, including the Devine formula for men and the Robinson formula for women. This web site also gives access to statistics such as the Metropolitan Life insurance tables of height and weight and much other useful information.[273]

Fat Deposit and Exercise

After diet correction, exercise is the next most powerful strategy for reducing body weight. We have certainly heard this before! But what we have not heard is that there are some provisos (stipulated conditions) we should be aware of that are rarely if ever mentioned by the promoters of exercise. The first proviso stems from the peculiar process by which energy is produced by our muscles. We have seen in chapter 2 that the body's ability to store glucose is very limited. What happens when you exercise? You are going to deplete your glucose storage. How do you feel after a workout? You feel great. You also may feel thirsty and hungry. Now comes the trick. If your next meal is loaded with carbohydrates you are simply going to refill your glucose storage sites and you are back at square one. However, if you combine your exercise with a low carbohydrate snack you will get two different consequences (the other two provisos).

First, your liver will be triggered to rebuild glucose molecules from the waste—the very waste products that accumulated as the glucose was being broken down and burned for fuel during exercise, i.e., lactate and pyruvate. This process of rebuilding glucose from waste products is energy intensive: it uses even more calories. Second, your cells will turn to fatty acids to meet their further energy needs. And where do these fatty acids come from? Stored body fat…the body fat that so many Americans have in such abundance, especially when we are highly overweight and obese.

Fat Deposit and Hormones

Fat storage and the depositing of excess fat in the body do not occur at random. Many hormones influence these processes: insulin, growth hormone, several steroid hormones (also known as corticoids) and thyroid hormone. Some of those hormones support the depositing of fat (insulin, corticoids, estrogens), whereas others oppose it (growth hormone, testosterone, thyroid hormone). Table 27 summarizes these hormone effects. As you will see in the table, the influence of all these hormones is selectively directed toward the accumulation of fat in different parts of the body.

	Insulin		Thyroid		Corticoid		Estrogen		Proges terone		Aldo steron		hGH		Testo sterone	
	+	-	+	-	+	-	+	-	+	-	+	-	+	-	+	-
Face	X			X	X					X				X		X
Neck				X			X			X				X		X
Shoulder						X										
Chest	X			X	X		X							w		X
Abdomen	X			X			X		w					X	w	m
Pelvis	X			X			X		X					X		
Thighs	X						X							X		X
Knee	X							X								X
Calf				X			X		X		X					
Ankle				X			X		X		X					

Table 27. List of some hormones and indication of their influence on fat deposit in various body locations. For each hormone a [X] in the columns under the sign [+] indicates the location of fat deposit triggered by an excess of that hormone. A [X] in the column under [-] indicates where fat most likely will accumulate in case of hormone deficit. The letter "m" and "w" indicate occurrence in men and in women respectively. Adapted from a lecture by Dr. Thierry Hertoghe MD. (hGH stands for human growth hormone.)

Estrogen in women, for example, supports fat deposition whereas the testosterone in men opposes fat deposition. Thyroid hormone deficiency supports fat deposition, while an excess of thyroid hormone opposes it.

The Leading Role of Insulin

Of all these hormones it is insulin that is of paramount interest to us for two reasons: (1) Insulin is the lead actor in human metabolism, and (2) the American diet is a repetitive drama of consistent and flagrant abuse of our insulin metabolism. If we eat the standard American diet we are in a protracted insulin crisis.

What and how much we eat is the domain of insulin. Indeed insulin is the only hormone whose activity is strongly influenced by food intake—more precisely, by the intake of sugar and starch. In chapter 3 we discussed how an excess of sugar and starch intake triggers and maintains abnormally high blood glucose and insulin levels. In this chapter we are coming to terms with the full ramifications of insulin's role as a storage hormone—causing the food we eat that is in excess of our immediate need to be stored as fat.

In essence, the excess of calories in the American diet is an excess of sugar and starch. Because of its effect on the hormone insulin it is the main factor in the overweight and obesity epidemic.

The Legacy of Overweight and Obesity

Overweight and obesity are not the real problem. Overweight and obesity are simply the external evidence, the indicators, that tell a generic story of excessive calorie intake. But they do not tell the inside story—that the real problem is usually too much starch and sugar consumed in the American diet. Too much starch and sugar keep the blood sugar level high (hyperglycemia). High blood sugar causes too much insulin to be released by the pancreas (hyperinsulinemia). And as we saw in chapter 4, high blood sugar and high insulin levels are responsible for the deterioration of blood vessels and the exaggeration of inflammatory and immune processes.

The health deterioration linked to overweight and obesity does not occur in adults only and it does not appear overnight. It may start in childhood in overweight and obese children. The consequences emerge anywhere from young adulthood to later in life in the form of hypertension, heart diseases, stroke, renal failure and an entire host of other ailments. Overweight and obesity also increase the risk of tumors, cysts and cancer. It is important to note that fat tissue is a source of potent hormone like substances and that fat accumulation results in too much of those products to be released. It is also important to note that these facts are only now coming to light and beginning to raise the concern they warrant.

What You Can Do

1. Reduce your intake of calories in the form of sugar and starch. This reduces your insulin level. Do it progressively. Your cells are tuned into glucose as their preferred fuel. Give them the time to switch to the best fuel, fatty acids.

2. Avoid stress. Stress increases the secretion of corticoids. As we have seen, corticoids are an additional factor in overweight and obesity in both men and women.

3. Seek the advice of a health professional. There is a high probability that you may have another hormonal imbalance in addition to too much insulin in your system.

Chapter 14

Wake up Americans!

Many things go better in the United States of America when Americans take matters into their own hands. And you have begun to do that.

You have read this book and learned that adaptation to environmental change is fundamental for all species to survive, that it takes time for adaptation to occur, and that lack of adaptation means suffering and premature death.

Now you know that our diet is an integral part of our environment, and you realize we have not had time to adapt to the environmental changes—the excesses and deficiencies—that the American diet has thrust upon us.

You are informed about the specific excesses of the American diet in the form of sugar and starch, omega-6 essential fatty acids, calories, pesticides and additives. You are equally informed about its deficiencies in the form of minerals and vitamins, omega-3 essential fatty acids, and key carbohydrates. You also are aware of the magnitude of the impact those excesses and deficiencies have on the health of all of us. If you haven't done it yet you should slide the CD into your computer and dig deeper into the information available on the Web concerning the topics of greatest interest to you.

You are well advised to correct your diet. This is a step you can certainly take on your own because you now know how you must proceed. However, if you are one of the 6 out of 10 Americans who is already experiencing diet-related health deterioration and you want to work with your physician to correct your diet and its consequences to your health, you need to know this: you may have to help her/him compensate for a lack of information. Medical schools do not teach the link between diet and health. They also ignore or deny the degree to which the American diet is responsible for a multitude of ailments. Provide your physician with a copy of this book or encourage him/her to order one at Amazon.com.

Aside from promoting the continuing education of your health professional so she/he can better help you recover from the American diet, you can also inform people around you of what you have learned. Do not underestimate your power to make a difference. The truth is that we will be educated by "the powers that be"—the food manufacturers, the multinational chemical corporations, the drug industry, and the media—or we will take matters into our own hands, open our minds to existing information and choose to prioritize our health above all else. It is especially important that this message reach politicians, regulators and other lawmakers. Encourage them to read this book and to browse the Web with the aid of the CD. They are in a position to correct existing rules and laws and to initiate new ones that may help alter the excesses and deficiencies of the American diet.

As Americans we are proud of our National Parks and of all the steps we take to protect the environment of endangered species. It may be time to add *Homo americanus* to this list of endangered species. Food is part of the environment of every living organism and the food environment of the Americans has been degraded in such a way as to endanger the survival of this species and to deteriorate the health of all.

Last but not least, be aware of this. The diet-related health decline of the American public costs our society hundreds of billions of dollars per year. These damages can be halted at a much lower cost and the money saved could be put to much, much better use.

Your comments and questions are welcome at *author@theamericandiet.com*

References

[1] *http://www.scirus.com*

[2] *http://www.longevinst.org/nlt/newsletter5ext2.htm*

[3] *http://www.longevinst.org/nlt/newsletter9ext2.htm*

[4] *http://www.cdc.gov/mmwr/preview/mmwrhtml/mm5126a 1.htm*

[5] *http://www.ncbi.nlm.nih.gov/entrez/query.fcgi?cmd=Retriev e&db=pubmed&dopt=Abstract&list_uids=10466159*

Comments:

A first flaw in the text is the claim that the actual prevalence of chronic diseases is related solely to dietary excesses. This claim totally ignores the fact that diet deficiencies are as important a factor in health as diet excesses. The author also confounds the vegetarian, Mediterranean and Asian diets, as if they were identical. The Mediterranean and Asian diets differ from the vegetarian diet in that they include the consumption of meat and fish. The author further pretends that the archeological record is insufficient to determine whether plants or animals predominated in the diet of our primitive ancestors. This 1999 claim ignores at least three previous publications demonstrating unequivocal evidence of meat and shellfish consumption by Paleolithic man.

[6] Blumenschine RJ, Cavallo JA, Scavenging and human evolution. In Scientific America 1992 Oct;267(4):90-6)

[7] *European Journal of Clinical Nutrition.* March, 2002. 56(Supplement 1):S42-S52.
Cordain, L.; Eaton, S. B.; Miller, J. Brand; Mann, N.; Hill, K. The paradoxical nature of hunter-gatherer diets: Meat-based, yet non-atherogenic.
http://www.ncbi.nlm.nih.gov/entrez/query.fcgi?cmd=Retrieve &db=pubmed&dopt=Abstract&list_uids=11965522

[8] *Journal of Archaeological Science.* Jan., 2000. 27(1):1-3. Richards, M. P.; Hedges, R.E.M.; Jacobi, R.; Current, A.; Stringer, C. Gough's. Cave and Sun Hole Cave human stable isotope values indicate a high animal protein diet in the British Upper Palaeolithic
http://www.sciencedirect.com/science?_ob=ArticleURL&_udi =B6WH8-45FC3DC-34&_coverDate=01%2F31%2F2000&_alid =223555799&_rdoc=1&_fmt=&_orig=search&_qd=1&_cdi=68 44&_sort=d&view=c&_acct=C000050221&_version=1&_urlVe rsion=0&_userid=10&md5=5f518bcd2deb12aa3ced5818a68e 7af4

[9] *Journal of Archaeological Science.* August, 2000. 27(8): 715-723. Hockett, Bryan Scott; Ferreira Bicho, Nuno. The rabbits of Picareiro Cave: Small mammal hunting during the Late Upper Palaeolithic in the Portuguese Estremadura.
http://www.sciencedirect.com/science?_ob=ArticleURL&_udi =B6WH8-45FC3951S&_coverDate=08%2F31%2F2000&_alid= 223556614&_rdoc=1&_fmt=&_orig=search&_qd=1&_cdi=684 4&_sort=d&view=c&_acct=C000050221&_version=1&_urlVe rsion=0&_userid=10&md5=e89bb5b59615ff24274e6dbd2a6 98736

[10] *Quaternary Research* (Orlando) Sept., 1997. 48(2):215-227. Serrano, Francisco; Guerra-Merchan, Antonio; Lozano-Francisco, Carmen; Vera-Pelaez, Jose. Multivariate analysis of remains of molluscan foods consumed by latest Pleistocene and Holocene humans in Nerja Cave, Malaga, Spain

[11] *Journal of Nutritional & Environmental Medicine* (Abingdon) 1996. 6(3):273-284. Teufel Nicolette I. Nutrient characteristics of Southwest Native American pre-contact diets.

[12] *Vegetation History and Archeobotany.* 1996. 5(1-2):33-38. Kubiak Martens Lucyna. Evidence for possible use of plant foods in Paleolithic and Mesolithic diet from the site of Calowanie in the central part of the Polish plain.

[13] *http://www.aces.uiuc.edu/~sare/columbian.html*

[14] *http://www.gluten.net/diagnosis.asp*

[15] *http://www.rpi.edu/dept/bcbp/molbiochem/MBWeb/mb 1/part2/sugar.htm*

[16] *http://images.google.com/images?q=glucose&ie=ISO-8859-1&hl=en&btnG=Google+Search*

[17] *Arabinose:*
http://images.google.com/images?hl=en&lr=&ie=ISO-8859-1&q=arabinose
Cellulose:
http://images.google.com/images?hl=en&lr=&ie=ISO-8859-1&q=cellulose
Fucose:
http://images.google.com/images?hl=en&lr=&ie=ISO-8859-1&q=fucose
Fructans:
http://images.google.com/images?hl=en&lr=&ie=ISO-8859-1&q=fructans&btnG=Search
Hemicellulose:
http://images.google.com/images?hl=en&lr=&ie=ISO-8859-1&q=hemicellulose&btnG=Search
Inositol:
http://images.google.com/images?hl=en&lr=&ie=ISO-8859-1&q=inositol
Insoluble fiber:
http://images.google.com/images?hl=en&lr=&ie=ISO-8859-1&q=insoluble+fiber
Inulin:
http://images.google.com/images?hl=en&lr=&ie=ISO-8859-1&q=inulin&btnG=Search
Invert sugar:
http://images.google.com/images?hl=en&lr=&ie=ISO-8859-1&q=invert+sugar&btnG=Search

Maltose:

http://images.google.com/images?hl=en&lr=&ie=ISO-8859-1&q=maltose&btnG=Search

Mannose:

http://images.google.com/images?hl=en&lr=&ie=ISO-8859-1&q=Mannose

Myoinositol:

http://images.google.com/images?hl=en&lr=&ie=ISO-8859-1&q=Myoinositol&btnG=Search

N-acetyl galactosamine:

http://images.google.com/images?hl=en&lr=&ie=ISO-8859-1&q=N-acetyl+galactosamine&btnG=Search

N-acetyl glucosamine:

http://images.google.com/images?hl=en&lr=&ie=ISO-8859-1&q=N-acetyl+glucosamine

Neuraminic acetyl acid:

http://images.google.com/images?hl=en&lr=&ie=ISO-8859-1&q=Neuraminic+acetyl+acid

Pectin:

http://images.google.com/images?hl=en&lr=&ie=ISO-8859-1&q=Pectin

Pentosan:

http://images.google.com/images?hl=en&lr=&ie=ISO-8859-1&q=%0DPentosan%0Dpentosan%0DPentosan%0D

Phytic acid:

http://images.google.com/images?hl=en&lr=&ie=ISO-8859-1&q=Phytic+acid

Raffinose:

http://images.google.com/images?hl=en&lr=&ie=ISO-8859-1&q=raffinose

Reducing sugar:

http://images.google.com/images?hl=en&lr=&ie=ISO-8859-1&q=Reducing+sugar

Sialic acid:
http://images.google.com/images?hl=en&lr=&ie=ISO-8859-1&q=sialic+acid
Soluble fiber:
http://images.google.com/images?hl=en&lr=&ie=ISO-8859-1&q=soluble+fiber
Sorbitol:
http://images.google.com/images?hl=en&lr=&ie=ISO-8859-1&q=sorbitol
Stachyose:
http://images.google.com/images?hl=en&lr=&ie=ISO-8859-1&q=stachyose&btnG=Search
Starch:
http://images.google.com/images?hl=en&lr=&ie=ISO-8859-1&q=starch
Sucrose:
http://images.google.com/images?hl=en&lr=&ie=ISO-8859-1&q=sucrose&btnG=Search
Trehalose:
http://images.google.com/images?hl=en&lr=&ie=ISO-8859-1&q=trehalose
Verbascose:
http://images.google.com/images?hl=en&lr=&ie=ISO-8859-1&q=verbascose
Xylitol:
http://images.google.com/images?hl=en&lr=&ie=ISO-8859-1&q=xylitol&btnG=Search
Xylose:
http://images.google.com/images/////////?hl=en&lr=&ie=ISO-8859-1&q=xylose*

[18] Glycogen:
http://images.google.com/images?hl=en&lr=&ie=ISO-8859-1&q=glycogen

Fructans:
http://images.google.com/images?hl=en&lr=&ie=ISO-8859-1&q=fructans&btnG=Search

[19] *http://www.GlycoScience.com/glycoscience/document_vi ewer.wm?FILENAME=D001*

[20] Wheat:
http://images.google.com/images?hl=en&lr=&ie=ISO-8859-1&q=wheat
Rice:
http://images.google.com/images?hl=en&lr=&ie=ISO-8859-1&q=rice
Barley:
http://images.google.com/images?hl=en&lr=&ie=ISO-8859-1&q=barley&btnG=Search

[21] Glucose:
http://images.google.com/images?hl=en&lr=&ie=ISO-8859-1&q=glucose%3A+&btnG=Search
Fructose:
http://images.google.com/images?hl=en&lr=&ie=ISO-8859-1&q=fructose
Galactose:
http://images.google.com/images?hl=en&lr=&ie=ISO-8859-1&q=galactose%3A+&btnG=Search

[22] Paleolithic diet:
Summary : *http://www.earth360.com/diet_paleodiet_balzer.html*
Full text at:
http://www.paleodiet.com

[23] Bill McAnalley, The Potential Significance of Dietary Sugars in Management of Osteoarthritis and Rheumatoid Arthritis: A Review. Proceedings of the Fisher Institute for Medical Research. Vol. 1, N°1, November 1997. 6-10.

[24] History of the recommendations of the U.S. Department of Agriculture (USDA):
http://iml.jou.ufl.edu/projects/Fall02/Greene/history.htm
Description of the food Pyramid
http://www.nal.usda.gov:8001/py/pmap.htm and
http://www.pueblo.gsa.gov/cic_text/food/food-pyramid/ main.htm
Outdated advice *http://www.ring.com/health/food/food.htm*

[25] *http://www.sucrose.com/lhist.html*

[26] *http://www.medical-library.net/sites/framer.html?/sites/_sugar_addiction.html*

[27] *Obes Res.* 2002 Jun;10(6):478-88. Evidence that intermittent, excessive sugar intake causes endogenous opioid dependence. Colantuoni C, Rada P, McCarthy J, Patten C, Avena NM, Chadeayne A, Hoebel BG. Department of Psychology, Princeton University, New Jersey 08544, USA.
http://www.ncbi.nlm.nih.gov/entrez/query.fcgi?cmd=Retrieve &db=PubMed&list_uids=12055324&dopt=Abstract

[28] *Factmonster* © 2002 Family Education Network 16 Jan. 2003: Sugar Consumption Skyrockets.
http://www.factmonster.com/ipka/A0779144.htm

[29] Sugar statistics:
http://www.cspinet.org/new/sugar_limit.html

[30] Sugar content of foods:
http://www.cspinet.org/reports/sugar/popsugar.html
Sugar economics:
http://ers.usda.gov/publications/agoutlook/mar1997/ao23 8g.pdf

[31] *Diabetologia.* 2001 Feb;44(2):129-46. "Advanced glycation end-products: a review. Singh R, Barden A, Mori T, Beilin L. Dept of Medicine, University of Western Australia and West Australian Heart Research Institute, Perth, Australia.
http://www.ncbi.nlm.nih.gov/entrez/query.fcgi?cmd=Retrieve &db=pubmed&dopt=Abstract&list_uids=11270668

[32] *http://www.clinidiabet.com/index_en.htm*

[33] *Life Sci* 2001 Jun 8;69(3):255-62. Short-term hyperglycemia induces lymphopenia and lymphocyte subset redistribution. von Kanel R, Mills PJ, Dimsdale JE. Department of Psychiatry, University of California at San Diego, La Jolla 92093, USA.
http://www.ncbi.nlm.nih.gov/entrez/query.fcgi?cmd=Retrieve &db=pubmed&dopt=Abstract&list_uids=11441916

[34] *J Clin Endocrinol Metab* 2001 Mar;86(3):1301-5 the article: Hyperglycemia acutely increases monocyte extracellular signal-regulated kinase activity in vivo in humans. Ceolotto G, Gallo A, Sartori M, Valente R, Baritono E, Semplicini A, Avogaro A. Department of Clinical and Experimental Medicine, University of Padova, 35100 Padova, Italy.
http://www.ncbi.nlm.nih.gov/entrez/query.fcgi?cmd=Retrieve &db=pubmed&dopt=Abstract&list_uids=11238524

210   *The American Diet*

[35] *Ann N Y Acad Sci* 2002 Apr;958:399-402. The lymphocyte as a cellular model to study insights into the pathophysiology of diabetes and its complications. Balasubramanyam M, Premanand C, Mohan V. the Madras Diabetes Research Foundation (MDRF), Gopalapuram, Chennai, India. *balusignal@hotmail.com*
http://www.ncbi.nlm.nih.gov/entrez/query.fcgi?cmd=Retrieve &db=pubmed&dopt=Abstract&list_uids=12021149

[36] *Immunol Lett* 2002 Jun 3;82(1-2):159-64. Effect of hyperglycemia on the basal cytosolic free calcium level, calcium signal and tyrosine-phosphorylation in human T-cells. Boldizsar F, Berki T, Miseta A, Nemeth P. Department of Immunology and Biotechnology, Faculty of Medicine, University of Pecs, Pecs, Hungary. *fboldizsar@hotmail.com*
http://www.ncbi.nlm.nih.gov/entrez/query.fcgi?cmd=Retrieve &db=pubmed&dopt=Abstract&list_uids=12008048

[37] *http://www.gsdl.com/assessments/fattyacids/appguide/index3.html*

[38] *Am J Physiol Heart Circ Physiol* 2002 Nov;283(5):H2130-9 Hyperglycemic switch from mitochondrial nitric oxide to superoxide production in endothelial cells. Brodsky SV, Gao S, Li H, Goligorsky MS. Department of Medicine, New York Medical College, Valhalla, NY 10595, USA.
http://www.ncbi.nlm.nih.gov/entrez/query.fcgi?cmd=Retrieve &db=pubmed&dopt=Abstract&list_uids=12384491

[39] *Circulation* 2003 Feb 25;107(7):1017-23. High glucose causes upregulation of cyclooxygenase-2 and alters prostanoid profile in human endothelial cells: role of protein kinase C and reactive oxygen specie. Cosentino F, Eto M, De

Paolis P,Van Der Loo B, Bachschmid M, Ullrich V, Kouroedov A, Gatti CD, Joch H, Volpe M, Luscher TF. Department of Cardiovascular Research, Institute of Physiology (F.C., M.E., B.v.d.L., A.K., C.D.G., H.J., T.F.L.), University of Zurich and Cardiovascular Center, University Hospital, Zurich, Switzerland.
http://www.ncbi.nlm.nih.gov/entrez/query.fcgi?cmd=Retrieve &db=pubmed&dopt=Abstract&list_uids=11063439

[40] *Diabetes* 2002 May;51(5):1556-64. Mechanisms of amelioration of glucose-induced endothelial dysfunction following inhibition of protein kinase C in vivo. Booth G, Stalker TJ, Lefer AM, Scalia R. Department of Physiology, Jefferson Medical College, Thomas Jefferson University, Philadelphia, Pennsylvania 19107-6799, USA.
http://www.ncbi.nlm.nih.gov/entrez/query.fcgi?cmd=Retrieve &db=pubmed&dopt=Abstract&list_uids=11978656

[41] *Med Klin* 2002 Apr 15;97(4):229-35. Atherosclerosis— progression by nonspecific activation of the immune system. Lehr HA, Sagban TA, Kirkpatrick CJ. Institut fur Pathologie der Johannes Gutenberg-Universitat Mainz.
lehr@pathologie.klinik.uni-mainz.de
http://www.ncbi.nlm.nih.gov/entrez/query.fcgi?cmd=Retrieve &db=pubmed&dopt=Abstract&list_uids=11977579

[42] *http://www.ncbi.nlm.nih.gov/entrez/query.fcgi?cmd= Retrieve &db=pubmed&dopt=Abstract&list_uids=14172263*

[43] *http://www.thincs.org/*

[44] *Neurochem Res* 2002 Nov;27(11):1341-7. Hyperglycemia triggers abnormal signaling and proliferative responses in Schwann cells. Almhanna K, Wilkins PL, Bavis JR, Harwalkar S, Berti-Mattera LN. Division of Hypertension, Department of Medicine, Case Western Reserve University School of Medicine, Cleveland, Ohio 44106, USA.
http://www.ncbi.nlm.nih.gov/entrez/query.fcgi?cmd=Retrieve &db=pubmed&dopt=Abstract&list_uids=12512939

[45] *http://www.ncbi.nlm.nih.gov/entrez/query.fcgi?cmd= Retrieve&db=pubmed&dopt=Abstract&list_uids=11522108*

[46] *Am J Physiol Cell Physiol* 2003 Jan;284(1):C200-8, the article: Inhibition of interferon-gamma expression by osmotic shrinkage of peripheral blood lymphocytes. Lang KS, Weigert C, Braedel S, Fillon S, Palmada M, Schleicher E, Rammensee HG, Lang F. Department of Immunology, University of Tubingen, Gmelinstrasse 5, D-72076 Tubingen, Germany.
http://www.ncbi.nlm.nih.gov/entrez/query.fcgi?cmd=Retrieve &db=pubmed&dopt=Abstract&list_uids=12475762

[47] *Diabetes Care.* 1989 Jan;12(1):56-61; discussion 81-2, Clinical aspects of sucrose and fructose metabolism. By Bantle JP. Endocrinology and Metabolism Department, University of Minnesota, Minneapolis.
http://www.ncbi.nlm.nih.gov/entrez/query.fcgi?cmd=Retrieve &db=pubmed&dopt=Abstract&list_uids=2653749

[48] *Physiol Res.* 2002;51(3):313-6. Advanced glycation end products and nutrition. Krajcovicova-Kudlackova M, Sebekova K, Schinzel R, Klvanova J. Institute of Preventive and Clinical Medicine, Bratislava, Slovak Republic *http://www.ncbi.nlm.nih.gov/entrez/query.fcgi?cmd=Retrieve &db=PubMed&list_uids=12234125&dopt=Abstract*

[49] Department of Medicine, the General Clinical Research Center, the Division of Biostatistics, and the School of Public Health, the University of Minneapolis, MN 55455, USA. *bantl001@tc.umn.edu*
http://www.ncbi.nlm.nih.gov/entrez/query.fcgi?cmd=Retrieve &db=pubmed&dopt=Abstract&list_uids=11063439

[50] *http://www.diabetes.ca/Section_About/timeline.asp.*

[51] *Autoimmun Rev.* 2003 Jun;2(4):204-10. Proinsulin-a pathogenic autoantigen in Type I diabetes. Narendran P, Mannering SI, Harrison LC. Walter and Eliza Hall. Institute of Medical Research, 1G Royal Parade, 3050, Parkville, Australia *http://www.ncbi.nlm.nih.gov/entrez/query.fcgi?cmd=Retrieve &db=pubmed&dopt=Abstract&list_uids=12848947*

[52] Gerald Reaven, M.D., is head of the Division of Endocrinology, Gerontology and Metabolism at Stanford University School of Medicine. He is also Director of the Geriatric Research, Education and Clinical Center at the Palo Alto Department of Veterans Affairs Medical Center. He has authored or co-authored more than 85 scientific articles that have appeared in peer-reviewed journals.

[53] *Diabetes.* 1988 Dec;37(12):1595-607. Banting lecture 1988: "Role of insulin resistance in human disease." Reaven GM. Department of Medicine, Stanford University Medical Center,California.
http://www.ncbi.nlm.nih.gov/entrez/query.fcgi?cmd=Retrieve &db=pubmed&dopt=Abstract&list_uids=3056758

[54] *Diabet Med* 1998 Jul;15(7):539-53. Definition, diagnosis and classification of diabetes mellitus and its complications. Part 1: diagnosis and classification of diabetes mellitus provisional report of a WHO consultation. Alberti KG, Zimmet PZ. Department of Medicine, University of Newcastle upon Tyne, UK.
http://www.ncbi.nlm.nih.gov/entrez/query.fcgi?cmd=Retrieve &db=pubmed&dopt=Abstract&list_uids=9686693

[55] *Curr Atheroscler* Rep. 2003 Sep;5(5):364-71. The insulin resistance syndrome. Reaven GM. Falk CVRC. Stanford Medical Center, 300 Pasteur Drive, Stanford, CA 94305, USA. *greaven@cvmed.stanford.edu*
http://www.ncbi.nlm.nih.gov/entrez/query.fcgi?cmd=Retrieve &db=pubmed&dopt=Abstract&list_uids=12911846

[56] *Nippon Rinsho.* 2003 Jul;61(7):1119-23. Hypertension and insulin resistance in obese Type II diabetic Wistar fatty rat. Suzuki M, Odaka H. Pharmacology Research Laboratories II, Takeda Chemical Industries, Ltd.
http://www.ncbi.nlm.nih.gov/entrez/query.fcgi?cmd=Retrieve &db=pubmed&dopt=Abstract&list_uids=12877072

[57] *Curr Diab* Rep. 2003 Aug;3(4):279-88. Molecular and physiologic actions of insulin related to production of nitric oxide in vascular endothelium. Vincent MA, Montagnani M, Quon MJ. Diabetes Unit, Laboratory of Clinical Investigation, NCCAM, National Institutes of Health, 10 Center Drive, Building 10, Room 6C-205, Bethesda, MD 20892-1632, USA. *quonm@nih.gov*
http://www.ncbi.nlm.nih.gov/entrez/query.fcgi?cmd=Retrieve &db=pubmed&dopt=Abstract&list_uids=12866989

[58] *Circulation.* 2003 Feb 25;107(7):1017-23. High glucose causes upregulation of cyclooxygenase-2 and alters prostanoid profile in human endothelial cells: role of protein kinase C and reactive oxygen species. Cosentino F, Eto M, De Paolis P, van der Loo B, Bachschmid M Ullrich V, Kouroedov A, Delli Gatti C, Joch H, Volpe M, Luscher TF. Department of Cardiovascular Research, Institute of Physiology, University of Zurich and Cardiovascular Center, University Hospital, Zurich, Switzerland. *f_cosentino@hotmail.com*
http://www.ncbi.nlm.nih.gov/entrez/query.fcgi?cmd=Retrieve &db=pubmed&dopt=Abstract&list_uids=12600916

[59] *Curr Diab* Rep. 2003 Jun;3(3):230-4, the article: Vascular compliance in diabetes. Winer N, Sowers JR. Division of Endocrinology, Diabetes, and Hypertension, Box 1205, SUNY Downstate Medical Center, 450 Clarkson Avenue, Brooklyn, NY 11203-2098, USA. *nwiner@downstate.edu*
http://www.ncbi.nlm.nih.gov/entrez/query.fcgi?cmd=Retrieve &db=pubmed&dopt=Abstract&list_uids=12762971

[60] *Nippon Rinsho.* 2003 Jul;61(7):1138-44. Higashi Y, Yoshizumi M. Department of Cardiovascular Physiology and Medicine, Graduate School of Biomedical Sciences, Hiroshima University.
http://www.ncbi.nlm.nih.gov/entrez/query.fcgi?cmd=Retrieve &db=pubmed&dopt=Abstract&list_uids=12877075

[61] *Curr Diab Rep.* 2003 Aug;3(4):293-8 Adipokines, inflammation, and the endothelium in diabetes. Aldhahi W, Hamdy O. Joslin Diabetes Center, One Joslin Place, Boston, MA 02215, USA. waleed.aldhahi@joslin.harvard.edu
http://www.ncbi.nlm.nih.gov/entrez/query.fcgi?cmd=Retrieve &db=pubmed&dopt=Abstract&list_uids=12866991

[62] *http://www.americanheart.org/presenter.jhtml? identifier=4718.*

[63] *http://www.signonsandiego.com/uniontrib/20040713/ news_1n13heart.html*

[64] *http://www.businessweek.com/magazine/content/04_30/ b3893048_mz011.htm* and
http://www.kansascity.com/mld/kansascity/news/nation/9 197133.htm?1c

[65] *http://www.signonsandiego.com/uniontrib/20040717/ news_1n17conflict.html*

[66] *Diabetes.* 2003 Aug;52(8):2160-2167. Prevalence and Characteristics of the Metabolic Syndrome in the San Antonio Heart and Framingham Offspring Studies. Meigs JB, Wilson PW, Nathan DM, D'Agostino RB Sr, Williams K, Haffner SM. Department of Medicine, General Medicine Division, Massachusetts General Hospital and Harvard Medical School, Boston, Massachusetts. Boston University School of Medicine and Framingham Heart Study, Framingham, Massachusetts. Diabetes Unit, Department of Medicine, Massachusetts Hospital and Harvard Medical School, Boston, Massachusetts. Department of Mathematics, Statistics, and Consulting Unit, Boston University, Boston, Massachusetts. Division of Clinical Epidemiology, Department of Medicine, University of Texas Health Science Center, San Antonio, Texas.

Abstract

http://www.ncbi.nlm.nih.gov/entrez/query.fcgi?cmd=Retrieve &db=pubmed&dopt=Abstract&list_uids=12882936

Full text

http://diabetes.diabetesjournals.org/cgi/content/full/52/8/2160

[67] *http://www.scirus.com/srsapp/sciruslink?src=web&url= http%3A%2F%2Farchsurg.amaassn.org%2Fcgi%2Fcollection%2 Fmetabolic_diseases%3Fnotjournal%3Darchsurg%2Camajnls*

[68] *Prog Cardiovasc Dis.* 2004 Jan-Feb;46(4):321-36. metabolic syndrome: An emerging health epidemic in women. Steinbaum SR.

http://www.ncbi.nlm.nih.gov/entrez/query.fcgi?cmd=Retrieve &db=pubmed&dopt=Abstract&list_uids=14961455

[69] Insulin and It's Metabolic Effect. The Crayhon Research Institute's BoulderFest August 1999 Seminar by Ron Rosedale MD.: *http://www.drbass.com/rosedale.html*

[70] *Eur J Clin Invest.* 2003 Dec;33(12):1051-69. Alterations in high-density lipoprotein metabolism and reverse cholesterol transport in insulin resistance and Type II diabetes mellitus: role of lipolytic enzymes, lecithin:cholesterol acyltransferase and lipid transfer proteins. Borggreve SE, De Vries R, Dullaart RP. Department of Endocrinology, University Hospital Groningen, Groningen, the Netherlands.
http://www.ncbi.nlm.nih.gov/entrez/query.fcgi?cmd=Retrieve &db=pubmed&dopt=Abstract&list_uids=14636288

[71] *Biochemistry.* 1991 Jun 4;30(22):5484-91. Solution structure of human insulin-like growth factor 1: a nuclear magnetic resonance and restrained molecular dynamics study. Cooke RM, Harvey TS, Campbell ID. Department of Biochemistry, University of Oxford, U.K.
http://www.ncbi.nlm.nih.gov/entrez/query.fcgi?cmd=Retrieve &db=pubmed&dopt=Abstract&list_uids=2036417
See the illustration of an insulin molecule at:
http://images.google.com/images?q=insulin&hl=en

[72] *Ann Endocrinol* (Paris). 2003 Jun;64(3 Suppl):S7-11. The diabetic pregnant woman. Lepercq J. Service de Gynecologie-Obstetrique, Hospital Saint-Vincent-de-Paul, F-75674 PARIS Cedex 14. *j.lepercq@svp.ap-hop-paris.fr*
http://www.ncbi.nlm.nih.gov/entrez/query.fcgi?cmd=Retrieve &db=pubmed&dopt=Abstract&list_uids=12910052

[73] *Am J Epidemiol.* 2003 Nov 15;158(10):963-8. Waist-to-hip ratio and breast cancer mortality. Borugian MJ, Sheps SB, Kim-Sing C, Olivotto IA, Van Patten C, Dunn BP, Coldman AJ, Potter D, Gallagher RP, Hislop TG. Cancer Control Research Program, British Columbia Cancer Agency, Vancouver, British Columbia, Canada. *mborugia@bccancer.bc.ca*
http://www.ncbi.nlm.nih.gov/entrez/query.fcgi?cmd=Retrieve
&db=pubmed&dopt=Abstract&list_uids=14607804

[74] *Endocrinol Invest.* 2003 Jul;26(7):683-5. Diabetic mastopathy: a case report. Giunta A, Vigneri R, Manusia M, Squatrito S, Tomaselli L. Divisione Clinicizzata di Endocrinologia e Dipartimento di Medicina Interna e Medicina Specialistica, Universita di Catania, Ospedale Garibaldi, Catania, Italy. *ariannagiunta@libero.it*
http://www.ncbi.nlm.nih.gov/entrez/query.fcgi?cmd=Retrieve
&db=pubmed&dopt=Abstract&list_uids=14594123

[75] *Br J Radiol.* 2003 Mar;76(903):192-4. Case report: diabetic mastopathy. Mak CW, Chou CK, Chen SY, Lee PS, Chang JM. Department of Diagnostic Radiology, Chi-Mei Foundation Medical Center, Tainan, Taiwan, Republic of China.
http://www.ncbi.nlm.nih.gov/entrez/query.fcgi?cmd=Retrieve
&db=pubmed&dopt=Abstract&list_uids=12684235

[76] *Chang Gung Med J.* 2003 Aug;26(8):540-53. Polycystic ovary syndrome (PCOS), insulin resistance and insulin-like growth factors (IGfs)/IGF-binding proteins (IGFBPs). Wang HS, Wang TH. Department of Obstetrics & Gynecology, Chang Gung Memorial Hospital, Taipei, Taiwan, ROC.
hswang86@ms17.hinet.net
http://www.ncbi.nlm.nih.gov/entrez/query.fcgi?cmd=Retrieve
&db=pubmed&dopt=Abstract&list_uids=14609034

[77] *J Biol Chem.* 2003 May 16;278(20):18063-8. Epub 2003 Mar 05. Microarray profiling of human skeletal muscle reveals that insulin regulates approximately 800 genes during a hyperinsulinemic clamp. Rome S, Clement K, Rabasa-Lhoret R, Loizon E, Poitou C, Barsh GS, Riou JP, Laville M, Vidal H. INSERM U.449 and Human Nutrition Research Center of Lyon, Faculty of Medicine R. Laennec, Lyon Cedex 08, France. *srome@univ-lyon1.fr*
http://www.ncbi.nlm.nih.gov/entrez/query.fcgi?cmd=Retrieve &db=pubmed&dopt=Abstract&list_uids=12621037

[78] *http://www.woundcare.org/newsvol1n3/ar1.htm*

[79] *Obes Res.* 1999 May;7(3):299-302. Dermatoses in 156 obese adults, by Garcia-Hidalgo L, Orozco-Topete R, Gonzalez-Barranco J, Villa AR, Dalman JJ, Ortiz-Pedroza G. Department of Dermatology, Instituto Nacional de la Nutricion Salvador Zubiran, Mexico City, Mexico.
http://www.ncbi.nlm.nih.gov/entrez/query.fcgi?cmd=Retrieve &db=pubmed&dopt=Abstract&list_uids=10348502

[80] *http://images.google.com/images?q=acanthosis+nigricans &ie=ISO-8859-1&hl=en*

[81] *Clin Pathol.* 2000 Nov;53(11):873-4. Comment in: J Clin Pathol. 2002 Aug;55(8):639; discussion 639. .Skin tags and the atherogenic lipid profile, by Crook MA. Department of Chemical Pathology, Guy's, St Thomas's, University Lewisham Hospital, London SE13 6LH, UK.
martin.crook@gstt.sthames.nhs.uk
http://jcp.bmjjournals.com/cgi/content/full/55/8/639-a

[82] *J. Dermatol.* 1995 Oct;22(10):729-31. Skin tags as markers of diabetes mellitus: an epidemiological study in India. Thappa DM. Department of Dermatology and STD, Jawaharlal Institute of Postgraduate Medical Education and Research (JIPMER), Pondicherry, India.
http://www.ncbi.nlm.nih.gov/entrez/query.fcgi?cmd=Retrieve &db=pubmed&dopt=Abstract&list_uids=8586750

[83] *http://images.google.com/images?q=keratosis+pilaris&ie= ISO-8859-1&hl=en*

[84] *http://images.google.com/images?hl=en&lr=&ie=ISO-8859-1&q=plantar+keratosis&btnG=Search*

[85] *http://images.google.com/images?hl=en&lr=&ie=ISO-8859-1&q=striae*

[86] *http://www.scirus.com/srsapp/search?q=metabolic+ syndrome&ds=jnl&ds=web&g=s&t=all*

[87] *Ethn Dis.* 2001 Fall;11(4):749-54. G6PD deficiency: its role in the high prevalence of hypertension and diabetes mellitus. Gaskin RS, Estwick D, Peddi R. Geriatrics Hospital, St. Michael, Barbados, West Indies.
http://www.ncbi.nlm.nih.gov/entrez/query.fcgi?cmd=Retrieve &db=pubmed&dopt=Abstract&list_uids=11763298
Comments: The genetic configuration described by Gaskin in 200 million people is not a genetic "defect," it is the original configuration. Our diet is defective not our genes.

[88] *http://www.lowcarb.ca/corpulence/corpulence_preface_1. html*
http://www.second-opinions.co.uk/banting.html

[89] *http://www.lowcarb.ca*

[90] *http://www.drsears.com/drsearspages/*

[91] *http://www.carbohydrateaddicts.com/*

[92] *http://www.eatprotein.com/*

[93] *http://forum.lowcarber.org/forumdisplay.php?f=52*

[94] Go to: *http://www.nerdheaven.dk/~jevk/paleo_intro.php* for information on the Paleolithic diet and comparison of the Paleolithic diet with other low carbohydrate diets.

[95] *http://www.second-opinions.co.uk/burn-fat.html*

[96] Read more at: *http://www.glycemicindex.com/main.htm* the home page of the glycemic index. See also GI related links at: *http://www.gisymbol.com.au/pages/links.asp*

[97] Read the full text and much more in a web page of the Food And Agriculture Organization of The United Nations at: *http://www.fao.org/docrep/w8079e/w8079e0a.htm# definition of glycemic index (gi)*

[98] *http://diabetes.about.com/library/mendosagi/ngilists.htm.*

[99] *http://ziag4.mmb.usyd.edu.au*, and enter a food name in the query box.

[100] Go to the web site of the National U.S. Library of Medicine at: *http://www.ncbi.nlm.nih.gov:80/entrez/query.fcgi* Entering the words "Glycemic Index" in the query box yields more than 600 publications.

[101] See the text of the petition introduced in 1999 to the FDA by the Center for Science in the Public Interest and requiring better sugar labeling on foods.

http://www.cspinet.org/reports/sugar/sugarpet1.pdf

The petition enumerates some reasons to reduce sugar intake: among them, the fact that excessive sugar intake increases the triglyceride level and favors obesity and tooth decay.

[102] *Harefuah*. 2001 Dec;140(12):1156-8, 1230. The effect of omega-3 fatty acids on risk factors for cardiovascular diseases. Yam D, Bott-Kanner G, Genin I, Shinitzky M, Klainman E. Weizmann. Institute of Science, Givatayim, Israel.

http://www.ncbi.nlm.nih.gov/entrez/query.fcgi?cmd=Retrieve &db=pubmed&dopt=Abstract&list_uids=11789299

[103] *Acta Diabetol*. 2002 Dec;39(4):209-13. Low serum magnesium levels and metabolic syndrome. Guerrero-Romero F, Rodriguez-Moran M. Research Group on Diabetes and Chronic Illnesses, Medical Research Unit in Clinical Epidemiology, Mexican Social Security Institute, Durango, Mexico.

Abstract

http://www.ncbi.nlm.nih.gov/entrez/query.fcgi?cmd=Retrieve &db=pubmed&dopt=Abstract&list_uids=12486495

Full text

http://www.springerlink.com/app/home/contribution.asp? wasp=7ped0mrutp5jpmxtwc2l&referrer=parent&backto=issue ,4,8;journal,13,41;linkingpublicationresults,1:100496,1

[104] *Scand J Clin Lab Invest.* 2000 Aug;60(5):403-9. Hyperglycaemia enhances renal magnesium excretion in Type I diabetic patients. Djurhuus MS, Skott P, Vaag A, Hother-Nielsen O, Andersen P, Parving HH, Klitgaard NA. Department of Clinical Biochemistry and Genetics, Odense University Hospital, Denmark.
http://www.ncbi.nlm.nih.gov/entrez/query.fcgi?cmd=Retrieve &db=pubmed&dopt=Abstract&list_uids=11003260
Read the information provided by the National Institutes of Health about magnesium at:
http://www.cc.nih.gov/ccc/supplements/magn.html#more
Visit the magnesium web site. It contains a huge list of links to magnesium-related web sites:
http://www.mgwater.com/list3.shtml and
http://www.mgwater.com/modern.shtml

[105] *Med Pregl.* 2000 May-Jun;53(5-6):319-24. Topalov V, Kovacevic D, Topalov A, Kovacevic D. Institut za kardiovaskularne bolesti, Sremska Kamenica, Medicinski fakultet, Novi Sad.
http://www.ncbi.nlm.nih.gov/entrez/query.fcgi?cmd=Retrieve &db=pubmed&dopt=Abstract&list_uids==11089379

[106] *BMC Public Health.* 2004 Nov 30;4(1):56. Mineral water intake reduces blood pressure among subjects with low urinary magnesium and calcium levels. Rylander R, Arnaud MJ. Department of Environmental Medicine, Sahlgrenska Academy at Goteborg University, Gothenburg, Sweden.
ragnar.rylander@envmed.gu.se
http://www.ncbi.nlm.nih.gov/entrez/query.fcgi?cmd=Retrieve &db=pubmed&dopt=Abstract&list_uids=15571635

[107] *J Nutr Biochem.* 2004 Dec;15(12):710-6. Magnesium deficiency and osteoporosis: animal and human observations. Rude RK, Gruber HE. University of Southern California and The Orthopaedic Hospital, Los Angeles, CA 90089-9317, USA.
http://www.ncbi.nlm.nih.gov/entrez/query.fcgi?cmd=Retrieve &db=pubmed&dopt=Abstract&list_uids=15607643

[108] *Ann Pharmacother.* 2003 Jun;37(6):876-85. Chromium as adjunctive treatment for Type II diabetes. Ryan GJ, Wanko NS, Redman AR, Cook CB. Department of Clinical and Administrative Sciences, Southern School of Pharmacy, Mercer University, Atlanta, GA 30341-4155, USA.
ryan_gj@mercer.edu
Abstract
http://www.ncbi.nlm.nih.gov/entrez/query.fcgi?cmd=Retrieve &db=pubmed&dopt=Abstract&list_uids=12773078
Full text
http://www.theannals.com/cgi/content/full/37/6/876

[109] *Clin Chem Lab Med.* 2003 Aug;41(8):995-8. Protective effects of antioxidant micronutrients (vitamin E, zinc and selenium) in Type II diabetes mellitus. Faure P. from the Laboratoire du Stress Oxydant et Pathologies Associees, Universite J. Fourier, Domaine de La Merci, La Tronche, Grenoble, France. *patrice.faure@ujf-grenoble.fr*
http://www.ncbi.nlm.nih.gov/entrez/query.fcgi?cmd=Retrieve &db=pubmed&dopt=Abstract&list_uids=12964803

[110] *http://www.nap.edu/pdf/0309069351/pdf_image/298.pdf* and following pages. Hint: to go to the following pages, enter the number of the page in the URL. Example: to go to page 299, the URL becomes:

http://www.nap.edu/pdf/0309069351/pdf_image/299.pdf Read the information provided by the National Institutes of Health about selenium at:

http://www.cc.nih.gov/ccc/supplements/selen.html

[111] *Am J Physiol.* 1992 Jan;262(1 Pt 2):R144-9. Sucrose-induced lipid, glucose, and insulin elevations, microvascular injury, and selenium. Lockwood MK, Eckhert CD. School of Public Health, University of California, Los Angeles 90024-1772.

Abstract

http://www.ncbi.nlm.nih.gov/entrez/query.fcgi?cmd=Retrieve &db=pubmed&dopt=Abstract&list_uids=1733334

Full text *http://ajpregu.physiology.org/cgi/reprint/262/1/R144*

[112] Professor G. N. Schrauzer has been actively involved in the development of nutritional selenium yeast supplements since 1976. He recognized the potential dangers of the misuse of selenium by manufacturers employing sodium selenite in place of genuine selenium yeast and wrote a letter to the FDA on April 25, 1978, in which he specifically warned about the possibility of widespread abuse of inorganic selenium compounds. During this period, Professor G. N. Schrauzer developed methods of distinguishing falsified supplements from the genuine organic selenium yeast products. One of his test kits is widely used by responsible manufacturers.

[113] *J Nutr.* 2000 Jul;130(7):1653-6., the article: Selenomethionine: a review of its nutritional significance, metabolism and toxicity. Schrauzer GN. Department of Chemistry and Biochemistry, University of California, San Diego, CA, USA. Abstract

http://www.ncbi.nlm.nih.gov/entrez/query.fcgi?cmd=Retrieve &db=pubmed&dopt=Abstract&list_uids=10867031

Full text *http://www.nutrition.org/cgi/content/full/130/7/1653*

[114] *Crit Rev Biochem Mol Biol*, 31(5-6):339-59 1996 Dec. Vanadium salts as insulin substitutes: mechanisms of action, a scientific and therapeutic tool in diabetes mellitus research: Sekar N; Li J; Shechter Y Department of Biochemistry, Weizmann Institute of Science, Rehovot, Israel.

http://www.ncbi.nlm.nih.gov/entrez/query.fcgi?cmd=Retrieve &db=pubmed&dopt=Abstract&list_uids=8994801

[115] *Journal of the American College of Nutrition*, 1998 Feb, 17(1):11-8. Verma S; Cam MC; McNeill JH. Nutritional factors that can favorably influence the glucose regulating system: vanadium.

[116] *Molecular and Cellular Biochemistry*, 1995 Dec 6-20, 153(1-2):205-9. Bhanot S; Michoulas A; McNeill JH. Antihypertensive effects of vanadium compounds in hyperinsulinemic, hypertensive rats

http://www.ncbi.nlm.nih.gov/entrez/query.fcgi?cmd=Retrieve &db=pubmed&dopt=Abstract&list_uids=8927040

[117] *Oncology Research*, 1999, 11(1):41-53. Bishayee A; Roy S; Chatterjee M. Characterization of selective induction and alteration of xenobiotic biotransforming enzymes by vanadium during diethylnitrosamine-induced chemical rat liver carcinogenesis. (UI: 99378239)
http://www.ncbi.nlm.nih.gov/entrez/query.fcgi?cmd=Retrieve &db=pubmed&dopt=Abstract&list_uids=10451030

[118] *Journal of Alternative and Complementary Medicine*, 1999 Jun, 5(3):273-91 Badmaev V; Prakash S; Majeed M. Vanadium: a review of its potential role in the fight against diabetes.. Pub type: Journal Article; Review; Review, Tutorial. (UI: 99308982)
http://www.ncbi.nlm.nih.gov/entrez/query.fcgi?cmd=Retrieve &db=pubmed&dopt=Abstract&list_uids=10381252

[119] *Biol Trace Elem Res.* 2003 May;92(2):173-80. Zinc supplementation attenuates thioacetamide-induced liver injury and hyperglycemia in mice. Song YM, Chen MD. Department of Medical Laboratories, Taichung Veterans General Hospital, Taichung, Taiwan.
http://www.ncbi.nlm.nih.gov/entrez/query.fcgi?SUBMIT=y
Read more about zinc at:
http://www.cc.nih.gov/ccc/supplements/zinc.html.

[120] *http://www.longevinst.org/nlt/newsletter19.htm*

[121] *Planta Med.* 2003 Jul;69(7):632-6. The antihyperglycaemic activity of berberine arises from a decrease of glucose absorption. Pan GY, Huang ZJ, Wang GJ, Fawcett JP, Liu XD, Zhao XC, Sun JG, Xie YY. Center of Pharmacokinetics, China Pharmaceutical University, Nanjing, China.
http://www.ncbi.nlm.nih.gov/entrez/query.fcgi?cmd=Retrieve &db=pubmed&dopt=Abstract&list_uids=12898419

[122] *http://www.nutrition.org/cgi/content/full/130/2/483S*

[123] *http://www.americanlongevity.net/company/wallach.php*

[124] *http://www.curezone.com/books/best/authorx.asp?ID=124*

[125] *International Journal for Vitamin and Nutrition Research.* Supp no. 27, 1985, pp. 61-73. "Concept of Borderline Vitamin Deficiency"

[126] *http://www.chiroweb.com/archives/21/03/13.html*

[127] *http://www.nal.usda.gov/fnic/dga/index.html*

[128] *http://www.longevinst.org/nlt/Vitamin_A_confusion.pdf*

[129] *http://www.longevinst.org/nlt/newsletter13ext1.htm #stearic*

[130] *http://www.longevinst.org/nlt/newsletter13ext1.htm#oleic*

[131] *http://www.ifst.org/hottop9.htm* is the web site of the United Kingdom Institute of Food Science and Technology (IFST), an independent professional qualifying body for food scientists and technologists. The IFST is totally independent of government, of industry, and of any lobbying groups or special interest groups.

[132] *http://diabetes.about.com/cs/newswire/a/blntransfats 903.htm*

[133] *http://images.google.com/images?q=fatty+acids&ie=ISO-8859-1&hl=en&btnG=Google+Search*

[134] *http://images.google.com/images?hl=en&lr=&ie=ISO-8859-1&q=phospholipids&btnG=Search*

[135] *http://images.google.com/images?hl=en&lr=&ie=ISO-8859-1&q=cell+membrane*

[136] *http://www.longevinst.org/nlt/newsletter13ext1.htm# linoleic*

[137] *http://www.longevinst.org/nlt/newsletter13ext1.htm#lino lenic*

[138] *http://www.cyberlipid.org/fa/acid0003.htm#3*

[139] *http://anatomy.utmb.edu/cellbio/membrane_intro.htm #Phospholipids*

[140] *http://images.google.com/images?hl=en&lr=&ie=ISO-8859-1&q=cells*

[141] *http://www.longevinst.org/nlt/newsletter13ext3.htm*

[142] Abstract:
*http://www.ncbi.nlm.nih.gov/entrez/query.fcgi?cmd=Retrieve
&db=pubmed&dopt=Abstract&list_uids=10617967*
Full text *http://www.ajcn.org/cgi/content/full/71/1/171S*

[143] A Scirus search yields more than 60,000 research papers on the essential fatty acid omega-3 published over the last 5 years. *http://www.scirus.com/srsapp/search?q=%28omega-3%29&cn=all&t=all&co=AND&q=&cn=all&t=all&g=a&fdt=2000&tdt=2005&dt=all&ff=all&ds=jnl&ds=web&sa=all&g=a*

[144] *http://lightsv.org/bud1.htm*
http://oradix.com/health/drjohannabudwigcancerdiet.shtml
Read about her books
1 - FLAX OIL AS A TRUE AID Against Arthritis, Heart Infarction, Cancer, at:
http://www.applepublishing.ca/index.cfm/book=288
2 - The OIL PROTEIN DIET COOKBOOK at:
http://www.applepublishing.ca/index.cfm/book=375

[145] The Omega-3 Essential Fatty Acids videos from the National Institutes of Health. To see the videos, you need RealPlayer basic that can be downloaded for free. (Go down to the end of the Real Player's page *http://www.real.com/* and click on the appropriate download icon.

1 - Conference by Bill Lands, Ph.D., Senior Advisor, NIAAA, NIH Overview of Essential Fatty Acids in Health and Disease. *http://videocast.nih.gov/ram/crii01c103202000.ram*
This talk notes how populations around the world have maintained certain food supplies in their surrounding

ecosystem and neglected others without considering the resulting impact on eicosanoid functions in their body. Informed food choices can supply the essential fatty acids that keep a balanced supply of eicosanoid precursors within the body to maintain balanced omega-6 and omega-3 eicosanoid responses of the body's inner ecosystem. **Comments**: Bill Lands introduces the fascinating and fruitful concept of the Inner Ecosystem.

2 - Conference by Norman Salem, Ph.D., Chief, Laboratory of Membrane Biochemistry and Biophysics, NIAAA, NIH Essential fatty acids- different chain lengths and metabolism. *http://videocast.nih.gov/ram/crii01c203202000.ram*
Norman Salem describes the structure and nomenclature for fatty acids for the non-specialist. He describes the chemistry and metabolism of omega-6 and omega-3 essential fatty acids to help people understand their nature in the context of more widely discussed saturated and unsaturated fats. The 18-carbon essential fatty acids can be metabolized to 20-carbon and 22-carbon forms that have different distributions in tissue membranes and have very different impacts on eicosanoid formation.
Comments: The conference by Salem covers in other words the topic described in chapter 9

3 - Eicosanoid formation, receptor functions, and clinical relevance by William L. Smith, Ph.D., Professor and Chairman of Biochemistry, Michigan State University
http://videocast.nih.gov/ram/crii01c303202000.ram
The talk describes the diversity of different eicosanoids that the body forms from the 20-carbon omega-6 and omega-3 essential fatty acids. This diverse set of hormone-like agents acts through different receptors on tissues to regulate many

different body responses in health and disease.

Comments: To follow this conference, one needs a background in biochemistry and physiology.

4 - *Essential fats in foods Penny Kris-Etherton, Ph.D., R.D., Professor of Nutrition, Pennsylvania State University*
http://videocast.nih.gov/ram/crii02c103202000.ram
This conference describes the amounts of omega-6 and omega-3 essential fatty acids present in many different foods currently consumed during typical food choices by the U.S. population. The talk presents food sources to help plan diets that meet target levels of omega-3 fatty acid intakes.

Comment: Practical recommendations.

5 - An overview of functional foods by Jean Pennington, Ph.D., R.D., Research Nutritionist, DNRC, NIH
http://videocast.nih.gov/ram/crii02c203202000.ram
The talk addresses the significance of the terms functional foods, designer foods, nutraceuticals and medicinal foods. The talk surveys different foods and lists the foods that contain the most functional components.

Comments: The author enumerates foods that contain active ingredients and what they do. This conference explains why the diet should contain a rich variety of vegetables and fruits.

6 - Differences between preventive nutrition and therapeutic intervention by Frank M. Sacks, M.D., Professor, School of Public Health, Harvard University
http://videocast.nih.gov/ram/crii02c303202000.ram
This talk describes principles involved in prevention and treatment interventions and notes the limitations in the types of evidence provided for forming personal decisions. Results

from several large diet therapy trials are reviewed to show benefits from selected diet interventions. There is definitive evidence that eating omega-3 fats decreases cardiovascular deaths. **Comments**: Sacks emphasizes that for official entities, innovative health guidelines are a low priority while historical uniformity and total security are imperative. One should not expect the latest health news from official agencies. The conference further highlights that in 1969 already the randomized Dayton trial had already proven that n-3 fatty acid supplementation reduces stroke by 43% and fatal heart attack by 31%.

[146] *http://www.longevinst.org/nlt/newsletter13ext3.htm#13-3-2*

[147] *JAMA* 2002 Nov 27,;288(20):2569-78. Optimal diets for prevention of coronary heart disease. Hu FB, Willett WC. Department of Nutrition, Harvard School of Public Health, 665 Huntington Ave, Boston, MA 02115, USA.
frank.hu@channing.harvard.edu
http://www.ncbi.nlm.nih.gov/entrez/query.fcgi?cmd=Retrieve &db=pubmed&dopt=Abstract&list_uids=12444864

[148] *http://www.whitehouse.gov/omb/pubpress/2003-13.pdf*

[149] All prompt letters as well as agency responses can be viewed at *www.omb.gov*

[150] *http://198.102.218.57/dietaryguidelines/dga2000/ document/images/pyramidbig.jpg*

[151] *http://www.cdc.gov/nchs/data/dvs/nvsr52_09p9.pdf*
and
http://www.cdc.gov/nchs/about/major/dvs/mortdata.htm

[152] *Chin Med J* (Engl). 2003 Mar;116(3):453-8., Omega-3 fatty acids and non-communicable diseases, Li D. Department of Food Science, Hangzhou University of Commerce, Hangzhou, 310035, China Email: *duoli@mail.hzic.edu.cn.*
http://www.ncbi.nlm.nih.gov/entrez/query.fcgi?cmd=Retrieve &db=pubmed&dopt=Abstract&list_uids=12781058

[153] *Am J Clin Nutr.* 2000 Jan;71(1 Suppl):224S-7S. n-3 fatty acids and the prevention of coronary atherosclerosis. von Schacky C. Medizinische Klinik, Klinikum Innenstadt, University of Munich, Germany.
vonschacky@medinn.med.uni-muenchen.de
http://www.ncbi.nlm.nih.gov/entrez/query.fcgi?cmd=Retrieve &db=pubmed&dopt=Abstract&list_uids=10617975

[154] *http://www.omega3ri.org/FDA.htm#HEffect*

[155] *http://www.medem.com/MedLB/article_detaillb.cfm? article_ID=ZZZW9JT7WHC&sub_cat=618*

[156] *Eur J Med Res.* 2003 Aug 20;8(8):337-54. N-3 polyunsaturated fatty acids and inflammation in the arterial wall. Yaqoob P, Calder PC. School of Food Biosciences, The University of Reading, Reading, UK. *P.Yaqoob@reading.ac.uk*
http://www.ncbi.nlm.nih.gov/entrez/query.fcgi?cmd=Retrieve &db=pubmed&dopt=Abstract&list_uids=12915325

[157] *Am J Clin Nutr.* 2003 Jul;78(1):65-71. Am J Clin Nutr. 2003 Jul;78(1):1-2. n-3 Fatty acids and 5-y risks of death and cardiovascular disease events in patients with coronary artery disease. Erkkila AT, Lehto S, Pyorala K, Uusitupa MI. Abstract

http://www.ncbi.nlm.nih.gov/entrez/query.fcgi?cmd=Retrieve &db=pubmed&dopt=Abstract&list_uids=12816772

Full text *http://www.ajcn.org/cgi/content/full/78/1/65*

[158] *http://www.ncbi.nlm.nih.gov/entrez/query.fcgi?cmd= Retrieve&db=pubmed&dopt=Abstract&list_uids=12848278*

[159] *http://www.cdc.gov/nchs/data/series/sr_10/sr10_200.pdf.*

[160] *Lancet.* 1998 Apr 25;351(9111):1225-32. Worldwide variation in prevalence of symptoms of asthma, allergic rhinoconjunctivitis, and atopic eczema: ISAAC. The International Study of Asthma and Allergies in Childhood (ISAAC) Steering Commitee.

http://www.ncbi.nlm.nih.gov/entrez/query.fcgi?cmd=Retrieve &db=pubmed&dopt=Abstract&list_uids=9643741

[161] *Allergy.* 2000 Aug;55(8):767-72. The prevalence of skin-test-positive allergic rhinitis in Danish adults: two cross-sectional surveys 8 years apart. The Copenhagen Allergy Study. Linneberg A, Jorgensen T, Nielsen NH, Madsen F, Frolund L, Dirksen A. Centre of Preventive Medicine, Department of Internal Medicine M, Glostrup Hospital, University of Copenhagen, Denmark.

http://www.ncbi.nlm.nih.gov/entrez/query.fcgi?cmd=Retrieve &db=pubmed&dopt=Abstract&list_uids=10955704

[162] From the American Academy of Allergy, Asthma and Immunology (AAAAI). The Allergy Report: Science Based Findings on the Diagnosis & Treatment of Allergic Disorders, 1996-2001.

[163] *http://www.aaaai.org/media/news_releases/2002/06/06 1102.html*

[164] *Ann Allergy Asthma Immunol.* 2004 Nov;93(5 Suppl 3):S12-8. Peanut allergenicity. Scurlock AM, Burks AW. Division of Pediatric Allergy and Immunology, Duke University Medical Center, Durham, North Carolina 27710, USA *http://www.ncbi.nlm.nih.gov/entrez/query.fcgi?cmd=Retrieve &db=pubmed&dopt=Abstract&list_uids=15562869*

[165] *http://www.ashp.org/latexallergy/index.cfm?cfid= 16408428&CFToken=32205147* and *http://www.users.globalnet.co.uk/~aair/latex.htm*

[166] *http://www.medscape.com/viewprogram/877_childindex*

[167] *http://www.lifespan.org/Services/Allergy/Articles/ insect.htm*

[168] *http://www.sfsu.edu/~shs/skinclinic/urticaria.htm*

[169] *http://ntri.tamuk.edu/immunology/autoimmunity.html*

[170] *http://www.Google.com*

[171] *http://www.niaid.nih.gov/dait/pdf/ADCC_Report.pdf*

[172] *http://www.asthmaworld.org*

[173] *http://www.asthmaworld.org/asthma_background.htm# Introduction.*

[174] *http://www.asthmaworld.org/pressrelease.htm#Dec 15* Read also how the CAPI, responding to a report by the National Academy of Sciences (NAS), brought into question the validity of the current direction of drug-based asthma research.
http://www.asthmaworld.org/pressrelease.htm#Dec.2

[175] *Am J Clin Nutr.* 2004 Sep;80(3):626-32. Fish intake is associated with a reduced progression of coronary artery atherosclerosis in postmenopausal women with coronary artery disease. Erkkila AT, Lichtenstein AH, Mozaffarian D, Herrington DM. Cardiovascular Nutrition Laboratory, Jean Mayer USDA-HNRCA, Tufts University, 711 Washington Street, Boston, MA 02111, USA.
http://www.ncbi.nlm.nih.gov/entrez/query.fcgi?cmd=Retrieve &db=pubmed&dopt=Abstract&list_uids=15321802

[176] *Ukr Biokhim Zh.* 2003 Jul-Aug;75(4):115-9. Related Articles, Links Effect of omega-3 polyunsaturated fatty acids on activity of glutathione-dependent enzymes in the liver cytosol and blood erythrocytes in rats with experimental chronic bronchitis and in the norm Korzhov VI, Zhadan VN. Yanovsky Institute of Tuberculosis and Pulmonology, Academy of Medical Sciences of Ukraine, Kyiv, Ukraine.
http://www.ncbi.nlm.nih.gov/entrez/query.fcgi?cmd=Retrieve &db=pubmed&dopt=Abstract&list_uids=14681984

[177] *Prim Care.* 2002 Jun;29(2):231-61. Related Articles, Links Respiratory and allergic diseases: from upper respiratory tract infections to asthma. Jaber R. Division of Wellness and Chronic Illness, Department of Family Medicine, University Hospital and Medical Center, Health Sciences Center, State University of New York at Stony Brook, Stony Brook, NY 11794-8461, USA.
rjaber@notes.cc.sunysb.edu
http://www.ncbi.nlm.nih.gov/entrez/query.fcgi?cmd=Retrieve &db=pubmed&dopt=Abstract&list_uids=12391710

[178] *Diabetologia.* 2004 Dec 29; Acute effects of monounsaturated fatty acids with and without omega-3 fatty acids on vascular reactivity in individuals with type 2 diabetes. West SG, Hecker KD, Mustad VA, Nicholson S, Schoemer SL, Wagner P, Hinderliter AL, Ulbrecht J, Ruey P, Kris-Etherton PM. Department of Biobehavioral Health, The Pennsylvania State University, University Park, PA, USA.
http://www.ncbi.nlm.nih.gov/entrez/query.fcgi?cmd=Retrieve &db=pubmed&dopt=Abstract&list_uids=15624100

[179] *Nutr Rev.* 2004 Sep;62(9):333-9. Polyunsaturated fatty acid regulation of gene expression. Sampath H, Ntambi JM. Department of Nutritional Sciences, University of Wisconsin, Madison, WI 53706, USA
http://www.ncbi.nlm.nih.gov/entrez/query.fcgi?cmd=Retrieve &db=pubmed&dopt=Abstract&list_uids=15497766

[180] *Clin Chem Lab Med.* 2003 Sep;41(9):1120-30. Diabesity: An inflammatory metabolic condition. Schmidt MI, Duncan BB. Graduate Studies Program in Epidemiology, School of Medicine, Federal University of Rio Grande do Sul, Porto Alegre, Rio Grande do Sul, Brazil.
http://www.ncbi.nlm.nih.gov/entrez/query.fcgi?cmd=Retrieve &db=pubmed&dopt=Abstract&list_uids=14598860

[181] *Chem Phys Lipids.* 2003 Nov;126(1):1-27. Docosahexaenoic acid: membrane properties of a unique fatty acid. Stillwell W, Wassall SR. Department of Biology, Indiana University Purdue University Indianapolis, 723 W. Michigan Street, 46202-5132, Indianapolis, IN, USA
http://www.ncbi.nlm.nih.gov/entrez/query.fcgi?cmd=Retrieve &db=pubmed&dopt=Abstract&list_uids=14580707

[182] *Pediatrics.* 2003 Jan;111(1):e39-44. Maternal supplementation with very-long-chain n -3 fatty acids during pregnancy and lactation augments children's IQ at 4 years of age. Helland IB, Smith L, Saarem K, Saugstad OD, Drevon CA. Institute for Nutrition Research, University of Oslo, Oslo, Norway. Peter Moller, avd Orkla, ASA, Oslo, Norway.
Abstract: *ingrid.helland@rikshospitalet.no*
http://www.ncbi.nlm.nih.gov/entrez/query.fcgi?cmd=Retrieve &db=pubmed&dopt=Abstract&list_uids=12509593
Full text:
http://pediatrics.aappublications.org/cgi/content/full/111/1 /e39

[183] *Psychiatr Clin North Am.* 2000 Dec;23(4):785-94. Docosahexanoic acid and omega-3 fatty acids in depression. Mischoulon D, Fava M. Depression Clinical and Research Program, Department of Psychiatry, Massachusetts General Hospital and Harvard Medical School, Boston, Massachusetts, USA.
http://www.ncbi.nlm.nih.gov/entrez/query.fcgi?cmd=Retrieve &db=pubmed&dopt=Abstract&list_uids=11147247

[184] *Dev Neurosci* 2000 Sep-Dec;22(5-6):474-80 The role of dietary n-6 and n-3 fatty acids in the developing brain. Innis SM. Department of Paediatrics, University of British Columbia, Vancouver, B.C., Canada.
sinnis@interchange.ubc.ca
http://www.ncbi.nlm.nih.gov/entrez/query.fcgi?cmd=Retrieve &db=pubmed&dopt=Abstract&list_uids=11111165

[185] *Altern Med Rev* 2000 Oct;5(5):402-28 Comment in: Altern Med Rev. 2000 Oct;5(5): 401. :Attention deficit/hyperactivity disorder (ADHD) in children: rationale for its integrative management. By Kidd PM.
http://www.ncbi.nlm.nih.gov/entrez/query.fcgi?cmd=Retrieve &db=pubmed&dopt=Abstract&list_uids=11056411

[186] *Am Acad Child Adolesc Psychiatry* 2002 Jul;41(7):799-805. Association of attention-deficit/hyperactivity disorder symptoms with levels of cigarette smoking in a community sample of adolescents. Tercyak KP, Lerman C, Audrain J. Department of Oncology, Lombardi Cancer Center, Georgetown University Medical Center, Washington, DC 20007-4104, USA. *tercyakk@georgetown.edu*
http://www.ncbi.nlm.nih.gov/entrez/query.fcgi?cmd=Retrieve &db=pubmed&dopt=Abstract&list_uids=12108804

[187] *Respiration* 2002;69(1):7-11. The neurobiology of tobacco dependence: a commentary. Balfour DJ. Department of Psychiatry, University of Dundee Medical School, Ninewells Hospital, Dundee, UK. *d.j.k.balfour@dundee.ac.uk*
http://www.ncbi.nlm.nih.gov/entrez/query.fcgi?cmd=Retrieve
&db=pubmed&dopt=Abstract&list_uids=11844955

[188] *Curr Opin Pediatr* 2002 Apr;14(2):219-23 . Abuse and toxicity of methylphenidate. Klein-Schwartz W. Research and Education, Maryland Poison Center and Department of Pharmacy Practice and Science, University of Maryland School of Pharmacy, Baltimore, Maryland 21201, USA.
wkleinsc@rx.umaryland.edu
http://www.ncbi.nlm.nih.gov/entrez/query.fcgi?cmd=Retrieve
&db=pubmed&dopt=Abstract&list_uids=11981294

[189] *J Child Adolesc. Psychopharmacol.* 2002 Spring;12(1):55-61 Methylphenidate-related growth impairment. Holtkamp K, Peters-Wallraf B, Wuller S, Pfaaffle R, Herpertz-Dahlmann B. Department of Child and Adolescent Psychiatry and Psychotherapy, Technical University, Aachen, Germany.
Kristian.Holtkamp@kjp.rwth-aachen.de
http://www.ncbi.nlm.nih.gov/entrez/query.fcgi?cmd=Retrieve
&db=pubmed&dopt=Abstract&list_uids=12014596

[190] *http://www.longevinst.org/nlt/newsletter13ext3.htm#13-3-2*

[191] *Rev Med Chil* 2001 Oct;129(10):1203-11. Docosahexaenoic acid (DHA) in fetal development and in infant nutrition. Valenzuela A, Nieto MS. Laboratorio de Lipidos y Antioxidantes, Instituto de Nutricion y Tecnologia de Alimentos, Universidad de Chile.
avalenzu@uec.inta.uchile.cl
http://www.ncbi.nlm.nih.gov/entrez/query.fcgi?cmd=Retrieve &db=pubmed&dopt=Abstract&list_uids=11775350

[192] *http://www.longevinst.org/nlt/newsletter13ext3.htm#13-3-2*

[193] *Pharmacological Research,* 1999 Sep, 40(3):211-25. Horrocks LA; Yeo YK.Health benefits of docosahexaenoic acid (DHA) [see comments].
http://www.ncbi.nlm.nih.gov/entrez/query.fcgi?cmd=Retrieve &db=pubmed&dopt=Abstract&list_uids=10479465

[194] *http://www.breastbabyproducts.com/postpartum depression.html*

[195] *J Affect Disord* 2002 May;69(1-3):15-29 Seafood consumption, the DHA content of mothers' milk and prevalence rates of postpartum depression: a cross-national, ecological analysis. Hibbeln JR. Laboratory of Membrane Biophysics and Biochemistry, National Institute on Alcohol Abuse and Alcoholism, National Institutes of Health, Park 5, Room 150, 12420 Parklawn Drive, 20892, Rockville, MD, USA
http://www.ncbi.nlm.nih.gov/entrez/query.fcgi?cmd=Retrieve &db=pubmed&dopt=Abstract&list_uids=12103448

[196] *http://www.thorne.com/townsend/dec/efas.html*

[197] *Pediatr Allergy Immunol.* 2004 Oct;15(5):442-8. Specific immunoglobulin E antibodies to peanut over time in relation to peanut intake, symptoms and age. van Odijk J, Bengtsson U, Borres MP, Hulthen L, Ahlstedt S. Department of Clinical Nutrition, Sahlgrenska Academy at Goteborg University, Gothenburg, Sweden.
http://www.ncbi.nlm.nih.gov/entrez/query.fcgi?cmd=Retrieve &db=pubmed&dopt=Abstract&list_uids=15482520

[198] *http://www.epa.gov/pesticides/biopesticides/ingredients/ factsheets/factsheet_011332.htm*

[199] *Curr Opin Clin Nutr Metab Care.* 2004 Mar;7(2):137-44. Alpha-linolenic acid metabolism in men and women: nutritional and biological implications. Burdge G. Institute of Human Nutrition, Biomedical Science Building, University of Southampton, Bassett Crescent East, Southampton SO16 7PX, UK. *g.c.burdge@soton.ac.uk*
http://www.ncbi.nlm.nih.gov/entrez/query.fcgi?cmd=Retrieve &db=pubmed&dopt=Abstract&list_uids=15075703

[200] *http://www.nutraingredients.com/news/ng.asp?id= 54818&n=dt264&c=sjkjsrqmkslqfvx*

[201] *Lancet.* 1993 Mar 6;341(8845):581-5. Intake of trans fatty acids and risk of coronary heart disease among women. Willett WC, Stampfer MJ, Manson JE, Colditz GA, Speizer FE, Rosner BA, Sampson LA, Hennekens CH. Channing Laboratory, Department of Medicine, Harvard Medical School, Boston, Massachusetts.
http://www.ncbi.nlm.nih.gov/entrez/query.fcgi?cmd=Retrieve &db=pubmed&dopt=Abstract&list_uids==8094827

[202] *J Nutr.* 2004 Apr;134(4):874-9. Trans fatty acids in adipose tissue and the food supply are associated with myocardial infarction. Clifton PM, Keogh JB, Noakes M. CSIRO Health Sciences and Nutrition, Adelaide BC, South Australia 5000. *peter.clifton@csiro.au*
http://www.ncbi.nlm.nih.gov/entrez/query.fcgi?cmd=Retrieve &db=pubmed&dopt=Abstract&list_uids=15051840

[203] *http://vm.cfsan.fda.gov/~dms/transfat.html*
and *http://www.cfsan.fda.gov/~dms/transfat.html#unhide*

[204] *http://napa.ntdt.udel.edu/trans/default.html*

[205] *http://www.glycoscience.com/glycoscience/home.wm*

[206] *Crit Rev Biotechnol.* 2002;22(1):65-84. Food-derived carbohydrates—structural complexity and functional diversity. Tharanathan RN. Department of Biochemistry and Nutrition, Central Food Technological Research Institute, Mysore, India.
http://www.ncbi.nlm.nih.gov/entrez/query.fcgi?cmd=Retrieve &db=pubmed&dopt=Abstract&list_uids=11958336
and
http://www.glycoscience.com/glycoscience/document_view er.wm?FILENAME=R001

[207] *http://www.longevinst.org/nlt/newsletter8ext1.htm#*

[208] *http://www.thorne.com/altmedrev/fulltext/osteo4-5-fig1.jpg*

[209] *http://www.aw-bc.com/mathews/MN/NACGALAS.GIF*

[210] *Annu Rev Biochem* 2003 Mar 27; *A Genetic Approach to Mammalian Glycan Function.* Lowe JB, Marth JD. Department of Pathology and HHMI, University of Michigan School of Medicine, Ann Arbor, MI 48109-0650.
http://www.ncbi.nlm.nih.gov/entrez/query.fcgi?cmd=Retrieve &db=pubmed&dopt=Abstract&list_uids=12676797

[211] *http://www.galab.com/technologies/glycosciences.html*

[212] *Science.* 2001 Mar 23;291(5512):2370-6. Glycosylation and the Immune System. Rudd PM, Elliott T, Cresswell P, Wilson IA, Dwek RA. The Glycobiology Institute, Department of Biochemistry, University of Oxford, South Parks Road, Oxford OX1 3QU, UK. *pmr@glycob.ox.ac.uk*
http://www.ncbi.nlm.nih.gov/entrez/query.fcgi?cmd=Retrieve &db=PubMed&list_uids=11269318&dopt=Abstract

[213] *Clin Immunol.* 1999 May;91(2):145-55. Neutrophilic myeloperoxidase-macrophage interactions perpetuate chronic inflammation associated with experimental arthritis. Lefkowitz DL, Gelderman MP, Fuhrmann SR, Graham S, Starnes JD 3rd, Lefkowitz SS, Bollen A, Moguilevsky N. Texas Tech University, Lubbock, Texas 79409, USA.
http://www.ncbi.nlm.nih.gov/entrez/query.fcgi?cmd=Retrieve &db=pubmed&dopt=Abstract&list_uids=10227806
Read more about the involvement of carbohydrates in inflammation at:
http://www.glycoscience.com/glycoscience/start_frames.w m?FILENAME=G004&MAIN=glyconutritionals&SUB=disease

[214] *http://www.tahoma-clinic.com/mannose.shtml*

[215] *http://www.nutritionalmedicine-wm.com/concepts.html*

[216] *http://www.glycoscience.com/glycoscience/start_frames.wm?FILENAME=D002&MAIN=glyconutritionals&SUB=introduction*

[217] *http://rics.ucdavis.edu/postharvest2/pubs/us_per_capita_cook.pdf*

[218] *http://www.who.int/dietphysicalactivity/goals/en/*

[219] *http://www.who.int/dietphysicalactivity/publications/facts/fruit/en/*

[220] *http://www.who.int/hpr/NPH/fruit_and_vegetables/lorelei.pdf*

[221] *http://lists.isb.sdnpk.org/pipermail/health-list/2003-January/002057.html.*

[222] *http://www.who.int/hpr/NPH/fruit_and_vegetables/ruth_bonita.pdf*

[223] *http://www.who.int/hpr/NPH/fruit_and_vegetables/pekka_puska.pdf*

[224] Consumption of fruits and vegetables in relation to the risk of developing acute coronary syndromes; the CARDIO2000 case-control study Demosthenes B. Panagiotakos, 1, 2 Christos Pitsavos, 1 Peter Kokkinos, 2 Christina Chrysohoou, 1 Manolis Vavuranakis, 1 Christodoulos Stefanadis, 1 and Pavlos Toutouzas 1. (1) Department of Cardiology, School of Medicine, University of Athens, Greece. (2) Veterans Affairs Medical Center and Cardiology Division, Georgetown University, Washington, DC, USA.
http://www.ncbi.nlm.nih.gov/entrez/query.fcgi?cmd=Retrieve &db=pubmed&dopt=Abstract&list_uids=12773206

[225] *http://www.mindfully.org/Pesticide/What-Is-A-Pesticide.htm*

[226] *http://www.mindfully.org/Food/Food-Additives-Definitions.htm*

[227] See the web site of the EPA at:
http://www.epa.gov/pesticides/regulating for more information.

[228] *Toxicol In Vitro*. 2000 Jun;14(3):227-34. Screening of selected pesticides for inhibition of CYP19 aromatase activity in vitro. Vinggaard AM, Hnida C, Breinholt V, Larsen JC. Institute of Food Safety and Toxicology, Division of Biochemistry and Molecular Biology, Danish Veterinary and Food Administration, Morkhoj Bygade 19, DK-2860 Soborg, Denmark. *amv@vfd.dk*
http://www.ncbi.nlm.nih.gov/entrez/query.fcgi?cmd=Retrieve &db=pubmed&dopt=Abstract&list_uids=10806373

[229] *Life Sci.* 1995;57(15):1433-40. Cytotoxic effects of post-harvest fungicides, ortho-phenylphenol, thiabendazole and imazalil, on isolated rat hepatocytes. Nakagawa Y, Moore GA. Department of Toxicology, Tokyo Metropolitan Research Laboratory of Public Health, Japan.
http://www.ncbi.nlm.nih.gov/entrez/query.fcgi?cmd=Retrieve &db=pubmed&dopt=Abstract&list_uids=7674834

[230] *http://www.businessweek.com/1996/19/b3474101.htm*

[231] *http://www.cspinet.org/reports/chemcuisine.htm#*

[232] *http://www.cfsan.fda.gov/~dms/eafus.html*

[233] *http://europa.eu.int/comm/food/fs/sc/scf/index_en.html http://www.foodstandards.gov.uk/news/newsarchive/aspar tamereview*

[234] *http://www.holisticmed.com/aspartame/scf2002.html*

http://www.foodandhealing.com/article-aspartame.htm

[235] *http://www.holisticmed.com/aspartame/abuse/seizures. html*

[236] *http://www.holisticmed.com/aspartame/abuse/migraine. html*

[237] *Cell Biol Toxicol.* 2002;18(1):43-50. Cytotoxic effects of methanol, formaldehyde, and formate on dissociated rat thymocytes: a possibility of aspartame toxicity. Oyama Y, Sakai H, Arata T, Okano Y, Akaike N, Sakai K, Noda K. Laboratory of Cellular Signaling, Faculty of Integrated Arts and Sciences, The University of Tokushima, Japan.
oyama@ias.tokushima-u.ac.jp
http://www.ncbi.nlm.nih.gov/entrez/query.fcgi?cmd=Retrieve &db=pubmed&dopt=Abstract&list_uids=11991085

[238] *http://www.scirus.com/srsapp/search?q=aspartame+ toxicity&ds=jnl&ds=web&g=s&t=all*

[239] *Pharmacol Sci.* 2003 Jan;91(1):83-6 Formaldehyde-induced shrinkage of rat thymocytes. Nakao H, Umebayashi C, Nakata M, Nishizaki Y, Noda K, Okano Y, Oyama Y. Laboratory of Cell Signaling, Faculty of Integrated Arts and Sciences, The University of Tokushima, Tokushima, Japan.
http://www.ncbi.nlm.nih.gov/entrez/query.fcgi?cmd=Retrieve &db=pubmed&dopt=Abstract&list_uids=1268673

[240] *http://www.cspinet.org/new/bromate.html*

[241] *http://www.oehha.ca.gov/prop65/pdf/noil_ABpkg19a1 a.pdf*

[242] *Chem Res Toxicol.* 2002 Aug;15(8):1106-12. Lung toxicity and tumor promotion by hydroxylated derivatives of 2,6-di-tert-butyl-4-methylphenol (BHT) and 2-tert-butyl-4-methyl-6-iso-propylphenol: correlation with quinone methide reactivity. Kupfer R, Dwyer-Nield LD, Malkinson AM, Thompson JA Department of Pharmaceutical Sciences, School of Pharmacy, University of Colorado Health Sciences Center, Denver, CO 80262, USA.
http://www.ncbi.nlm.nih.gov/entrez/query.fcgi?cmd=Retrieve&db=pubmed&dopt=Abstract&list_uids=12184795

[243] *J Paediatr Child Health.* 2002 Aug;38(4):373-6. Controlled trial of cumulative behavioral effects of a common bread preservative. Dengate S., Ruben A. *sdengate@ozemail.com.au http://www.ncbi.nlm.nih.gov/entrez/query.fcgi?cmd=Retrieve&db=pubmed&dopt=Abstract&list_uids=12173999*

[244] *http://risk.lsd.ornl.gov/tox/profiles/sulfate_f_V1.shtml*

[245] *http://www.hacsg.org.uk/*

[246] *http://www.texturant systems.com/texturant/html/e/products/carra.htm*
See a drawing of carrageenans at
http://www.lsbu.ac.uk/water/hycar.html

[247] *http://allergies.about.com/od/inulin/*

[248] *http://sci-toys.com/ingredients/maltitol.html*

[249] *http://www.holisticmed.com/msg/msg-mark.txt*

[250] A summary of the book "Exitotoxins, the Taste that Kills"
from Dr. Blaylock is available at:
http://members.aol.com/ICRelief/msgaspartame.html
Read an interview of Dr Blaylock MD about the effect of
additives on brain and brain function at
http://www.holisticmed.com/add/blaylock.html

[251] *http://users.ox.ac.uk/~trin0992/life/pepper.htm*

[252] *http://www.cspinet.org/sodapop/liquid_candy.htm*

[253] *http://www.kauhawaii.com/softdrinks.html*

[254] *http://cis.nci.nih.gov/fact/3_19.htm*

[255] *http://www.rense.com/general/nutrano.htm*

[256] *http://sci-toys.com/ingredients/sucralose.html*

[257] *http://www.splenda.com/page.jhtml?id=splenda/products/
faq.inc*

[258] *http://www.mercola.com/2000/dec/3/sucralose_
product.htm*
http://www.mercola.com/2000/dec/3/sucralose_dangers.htm

[259] *http://consumerlawpage.com/article/gulfwar.shtml*

[260] *http://www.gastronomique.org/*

[261] *http://health.discovery.com/tools/calculators/basal/
basal.html*

[262] *http://web.mawebcenters.com/gpindustries4/daily calorieneeds.ivnu*

[263] *http://www.apexfitness.com/html/tools/fit_calc/calorie/*

[264] *Psychol Sci.* 2003 Sep;14(5):450-4. The ecology of eating: smaller portion sizes in France than in the United States help explain the French paradox. Rozin P, Kabnick K, Pete E, Fischler C, Shields C. University of Pennsylvania and CNRS, Paris, France. *rozin@psych.upenn.edu*
http://www.ncbi.nlm.nih.gov/entrez/query.fcgi?cmd=Retrieve &db=pubmed&dopt=Abstract&list_uids=12930475

[265] The Contribution of Expanding Portion Sizes to the U.S. Obesity Epidemic Lisa R. Young, PhD, RD and Marion Nestle, PhD, MPH. Department of Nutrition and Food Studies, New York University, New York City. Correspondence: Requests for reprints should be sent to Lisa R. Young, PhD, RD, Department of Nutrition and Food Studies, New York University, 35 W 4th St, 10th Floor, New York, NY 10012-1172 (e-mail: *lisa.young@nyu.edu*)
http://www.ncbi.nlm.nih.gov/entrez/query.fcgi?cmd=Retrieve &db=pubmed&dopt=Abstract&list_uids=11818300
http://www.ncbi.nlm.nih.gov/entrez/query.fcgi?cmd=Retrieve &db=pubmed&dopt=Abstract&list_uids=11818300

[266] *JAMA.* 1994 Jul 20;272(3):205-11. Increasing prevalence of overweight among US adults. The National Health and Nutrition Examination Surveys, 1960 to 1991. Kuczmarski RJ, Flegal KM, Campbell SM, Johnson CL. Division of Health Examination Statistics, Centers for Disease Control and Prevention, Hyattsville, MD.
http://www.ncbi.nlm.nih.gov/entrez/query.fcgi?cmd=Retrieve&db=pubmed&dopt=Abstract&list_uids=8022039

[267] *JAMA.* 2002 Oct 9;288(14):1723-7. Prevalence and trends in obesity among US adults, 1999-2000. Flegal KM, Carroll MD, Ogden CL, Johnson CL.National Center for Health Statistics, 6525 Belcrest Rd, Room 900, Hyattsville, MD 20782, USA. kmf2@cdc.gov
http://www.ncbi.nlm.nih.gov/entrez/query.fcgi?cmd=Retrieve&db=pubmed&dopt=Abstract&list_uids=12365955

[268] Morbidity and Mortality Weekly Report; 2/6/2004; Johnson, CL Division of Health Examination Statistics, Centers for Disease Control and Prevention, Hyattsville, MD

[269] *JAMA.* 2002 Oct 9;288(14):1723-t. Prevalence and trends in obesity among US adults, 1999-2000. Flegal KM, Carroll MD, Ogden CL, Johnson CL.Center for Health Statistics, 6525 Belcrest Rd, Room 900, Hyattsville, MD 20782, USA. *kmf2@cdc.gov kmf2@cdc.gov*
http://www.ncbi.nlm.nih.gov/entrez/query.fcgi?cmd=Retrieve&db=pubmed&dopt=Abstract&list_uids=12365955

[270] *http://nhlbisupport.com/bmi/bmicalc.htm*
http://www.prescriptiondrugs.com/calculator.htm?a=p&b=25-10

[271] *http://www.cdc.gov/nccdphp/dnpa/bmi/bmi-adult-formula.htm*

[272] *http://www.halls.md/ideal-weight/body.htm*

[273] *http://www.halls.md/mapit.htm*